TALKING

sexuality
safety
reproduction
diversity
health
consent
pleasure
bodies
positivity
relationships

...SEX & more

A conversation guide for parents

VANESSA HAMILTON

amba
press

Copyright © Vanessa Hamilton 2023

All rights reserved. No part of this book may be reproduced or transmitted in any form or by any means, electronic or mechanical, including photocopying, recording or by any information storage and retrieval system, without prior permission in writing from the publisher.

Published in 2023 by Amba Press, Melbourne, Australia
www.ambapress.com.au

Editor - Brooke Lyons
Cover and internal designer - Tess McCabe

ISBN: 9781922607782 (pbk)
ISBN: 9781922607799 (ebk)

A catalogue record for this book is available from the National Library of Australia.

Content warning

Many people's experiences of sex and sexuality are not positive ones. On any given day we may not feel up to thinking about these topics. Please lean in to how you are feeling. Take a break if you need to.

This book includes discussion of topics such as sexual violence and child sexual abuse. If you find these topics challenging, please consider accessing professional care and support. You deserve to have help and understanding around any trauma or adverse experiences no matter how long ago they occurred.

Pick up the phone to your local support services or see the Resources section of this book for information suggestions. For many this will be a brave first step; however, especially if you are a parent, some healing around this will likely benefit both you and potentially your children.

Take care.

A note on language

In this book I'll tell you why I don't like the word 'sex', why it is mostly unhelpful and why I hardly ever use it when I educate. I can't avoid using the word 'sex' in this book altogether, though, as it does have some (very limited) practicality, such as being the simplest word most people relate to and understand. I hope to change that with this book – to open your minds to language that is more specific, expansive, inclusive and respectful rather than inaccurately using 'sex' for everything.

When I say 'children' this broadly refers to those aged 17 years and under. At times I will use more age-specific terms. Children learn in different ways at unique ages and stages. The information is intended for you to adapt to the circumstances of your child's learning ability, taking into account disability, learning challenges and language.

The term 'parents' also implies primary carers.

This book is grounded in Western cultural practices. Please make space for your own values, faith, culture and opinions.

Contents

Introduction   1

Chapter 1 — The basics of sexuality education   10

Chapter 2 — Conversations, ages and stages   29

Chapter 3 — Reproduction   50

Chapter 4 — Puberty   60

Chapter 5 — Human sexuality diversity   69

Chapter 6 — Sexual wellbeing in the digital age   96

Chapter 7 — Respect, consent and sexual violence   114

Final thoughts: top 20 tips   146

Sexuality conversation starters   156

Resources   162

References   165

About Vanessa   171

Acknowledgements   173

The aim of this book is to help you become the askable and tellable adult that children need you to be.

Let's get started - it's easier than you think.

Introduction

'Mum, how does the man stop the wee from coming out when he is putting the seed in the vagina?'

Would you know how to answer this question, from a five-year-old? I didn't – even though, at the time, I was a sexual and reproductive health nurse with more than 15 years' experience, and a university lecturer in human sexuality! I'd literally had tens of thousands of conversations about sex and sexuality, including the basics with my kids, but I still wasn't prepared for my young son's question. In that moment I realised my clinical and educator experience hadn't prepared me to talk to little kids about this topic, let alone tackle the complex parental responsibility of having conversations about sexuality with my older children one day. And if I was struggling, how did parents *without* my knowledge have any chance of meeting their kids' needs?

That insightful question from my son, 13 years ago, led me to start my business: Talking the Talk Healthy Sexuality Education. I have had the absolute privilege of teaching sexuality education ('sex ed') in schools and universities at all year levels, ages five to 21, and now focus on teaching and supporting educators, parents and carers.

Why read this book?

Your children are getting a sexuality education every day from the world around them. But is it the one you want them to receive?

I have written this book to help you have important conversations with your kids about sex, or more accurately: human sexuality, respectful relationships and consent. I like to call it HSRRC.

Whether you like it or not, HSRRC education is your children's right and your responsibility. One of your most important accountabilities as a parent is to be the main, trusted source of comprehensive, age-appropriate information, giving children the best opportunity for a safe, healthy and happy journey through life.

After more than 25 years working in sexual health at organisations including Kobler Centre London, Melbourne Sexual Health Centre and Austin Health Melbourne, and educating postgraduate students at the University of Melbourne, I decided to dedicate the next phase of my professional life to the current generation of children. My aim is to empower them with the essential education and tools they need for safe and positive development and relationship experiences – and to support as many adults as I can to be the main source of HSRRC information for children.

We have to ensure that children's basic human right to knowledge is upheld via education that supports age-appropriate development and wellbeing for a lifetime. HSRRC education underpins a deep and empowered sense of self, as well as helping children foster relationships and experiences that are respectful, fulfilling, enriching, pleasurable, joyful, healthy and safe. According to UNESCO (2018), comprehensive and accurate human sexuality education can:

- increase adolescents' confidence and ability to make informed decisions
- encourage respect, acceptance, equality and empathy
- delay the initiation of sexual intercourse to a later age
- help young people to distinguish between accurate and inaccurate information found online
- help prevent sexual abuse
- increase the use of contraception
- prevent unintended pregnancy and sexually transmitted infections (STIs)
- provide additional opportunities for young people to learn about and discuss relationships and sexual health issues outside their homes.

It's also strongly supported by the majority of parents (Hendriks et al. 2023).

How will you ensure you are the first person to educate your children about HSRRC, before the media, advertising, popular culture, porn, online games, the internet and the schoolyard? When will you need to begin in order to be the first to tell them about each topic?

In my experience, most parents feel unprepared for these conversations, and uninformed by their own sexuality education experience – and therefore lack confidence in their ability to meet their children's needs for knowledge around sexual health and wellbeing. Many adults tell me they never received adequate or accurate information around sexuality and relationships, yet they find themselves responsible for their own children's sexual health, wellbeing and safety. They know they must provide their children with adequate, accurate information in a positive and useful way, but they're not sure how to go about it, or when to start.

Many adults were brought up to believe these topics were not 'safe' to talk about. There may have been hushed tones or a complete lack of discussion, even about the basics of puberty. In most cases there was certainly no mention of pleasurable and consensual experiences or intimacy in relationships. We commonly carry that shame, fear and taboo, and resulting embarrassment, into our adult relationships. Many of us lack the ability to converse about these topics with our adult sexual partners, let alone talk to children about them. Parents play the biggest role in, and have the greatest influence over, this aspect of health, safety and wellbeing, yet important opportunities to make a difference are often missed.

I wrote this book to support you in having these essential, life-altering conversations with your children. My aim is to dispel the myths, misinformation and fears I hear from adults time and time again. Along with my professional knowledge I'll share stories of my own experiences and those of other parents. You might recognise some of them as resembling your experiences; I often hear very similar stories from multiple adults. I have changed details in all of the stories to protect privacy.

I hope this book provides information and answers you never received yourself. However, this is not a textbook. I have described the very basics of the key topics in simplified language and provided resources so you can dive in deeper if you want to. I've also included conversation starters, scripts for answering curly questions, opportunities for self-reflection and suggested topics you should research further for your family conversations.

Who do you want to tell your child about each topic related to sex, human sexuality, consent and respect?

Who do you want to be the main provider of this information?

*Hopefully the answer is **you**.*

If so, when do you need to start to ensure you get in first?

Throughout these chapters I offer my thoughts, opinions and examples based on my knowledge and experience, current research and contemporary literature, and the tens of thousands of conversations I've had with adults and children about sexuality. I also give you contemporary alternatives to the language we currently use that no longer serves us (and often never did). However, all families and experiences are diverse, so please make space for your own opinions, values, parenting styles, faith, culture and judgements. At times you may disagree, but let's respect others' opinions, especially when publicly commenting online.

I hope you'll find the book to be a simple guide that empowers you to support your kids to write their own unique version of their sexuality script for life. After all, sexuality is a core aspect of being human, from birth to death. I acknowledge that it is a huge shift to reject embedded, pervasive sexuality scripts and gender norms, but global evidence points to the benefit of rethinking these unhelpful and often harmful discourses. Our children deserve better, and we must get started and turn these inaccurate and damaging expectations around.

Congratulations on making the effort to access this book. I invite you to be expansive and open in your thinking and learning as you go through it.

After all, there is one thing we can all agree on: ensuring the health, safety and wellbeing of children.

Answering the curly questions

At this point you may be wondering, what *did* I tell my five-year-old son when he essentially asked me about orgasm and ejaculation? Well, the best response I could come up with on the spot was, 'He does a wee first.' Which is sort of, partly, not really correct!

Five years later my son came home late from sport and was eating his dinner while I sat with my laptop, preparing my slide presentation for the parent session I was running at his primary school. He said, 'Mum, what is on your first slide? What do you say to get them interested?' I'd been meaning to get his consent to use the question he had asked as a five-year-old, so this was the perfect opportunity.

I said, 'I tell them a story of a five-year-old asking his mum how the man stops the wee from coming out when he is putting the seed in the vagina.' My son replied, 'Oh, good question. I know! He does a wee first!' I kid you not: he remembered!

We went on to have a deeper age-appropriate conversation about the brain being the most important sexual organ, and how it sends a message to the bladder to block off so that only one fluid passes through and out of the urethra at a time.

Thinking about your parenting style, how would you have answered this question from a five-year-old? Perhaps you'll have some more ideas once you continue through this book.

Change is uncomfortable, but it is necessary. Parents are key to the next generation's lifelong health, happiness and wellbeing in regards to their sexuality. This is an opportunity to expand your learning and increase your skills for a better future for our kids. It is possible, and I hope this book makes a difference.

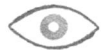 Self-reflection

- Thinking back, how did you learn about this thing called 'sex'? What do you wish you had been taught about sexuality and relationships when you were growing up?
- What age are your children? What sexuality education have they had so far?
- Where do your children currently get their sexuality messages from?
  - ☐ Me
  - ☐ Other parent(s)
  - ☐ Other carers
  - ☐ Family members
  - ☐ School classroom
  - ☐ School playground
  - ☐ Friends/peers
  - ☐ Pornography
  - ☐ Social media (TikTok, Instagram, Snapchat)
  - ☐ Society
  - ☐ TV
  - ☐ Advertising
  - ☐ Music videos
  - ☐ Books
  - ☐ I don't know
  - ☐ Other

- Where do you want your children to get their sexuality messages from?
    - ☐ Me
    - ☐ Other parent(s)
    - ☐ Other carers
    - ☐ Family members
    - ☐ School classroom
    - ☐ School playground
    - ☐ Friends/peers
    - ☐ Pornography
    - ☐ Social media (TikTok, Instagram, Snapchat)
    - ☐ Society
    - ☐ TV
    - ☐ Advertising
    - ☐ Music videos
    - ☐ Books
    - ☐ I don't know
    - ☐ Other
- When your child is an adult, how do you want them to describe their learning about these topics and your parenting around them?
- When you hear the word 'sex', what do you think it means?

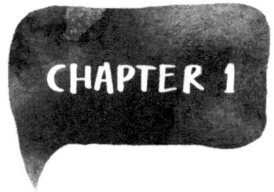

CHAPTER 1

The basics of sexuality education

What the #*%! does 'sex' mean, anyway?

When I present to parents, teachers and health professionals, I ask them, 'What do people in our society broadly think of when they hear the word 'sex'?' We always come up with two main interpretations of this word:

1. Heterosexual penis-in-vagina intercourse (responses often include things like 'the act of', 'doing it', 'the deed', 'the physical act', 'intercourse' and so on)

2. Being male or female (responses always include 'gender').

In reality, the word 'sex' means different things to different people. The focus on penis-in-vagina heterosexual intercourse as the most important part of ideal sexual function and that sex is only male or female is really unhelpful. Heterosexual intercourse is such a small component of human sexuality, yet it is often the biggest barrier preventing conversations from getting started! The inaccurate concept of the binary division of only male or female is also very limiting compared to what we actually know about the breadth, complexity, diversity, development, behaviour and uniqueness of each person's sexuality journey through life. The necessary education and essential conversations regarding human sexuality actually have hardly anything to do with what people commonly think of when they hear the word 'sex'. I especially dislike the term 'sex education' as it implies that we are only talking about the act of sex, and/or the harmful binary discourse that humans must fit into one of two boxes as far as their sexuality is concerned.

As I mentioned in the introduction, my preference is to use the term 'HSRRC' – human sexuality, respectful relationships and consent.

The World Health Organization (2023a) describes sexual health as follows:

- *About wellbeing, not merely the absence of disease*
- *Involves respect, safety and freedom from discrimination and violence*
- *Depends on the fulfilment of certain human rights*
- *Expressed through diverse sexualities and forms of sexual expression*
- *Is critically influenced by gender norms, roles, expectations and power dynamics*
- *Needs to be understood within specific social, economic and political contexts.*

The following definition of sexuality from the World Health Organization (2017) is what we need to be teaching children (not just 'sex'):

Sexuality is a central aspect of being human throughout life and encompasses sex, gender identities and roles, sexual orientation, eroticism, pleasure, intimacy and reproduction.

> *Sexuality is influenced by the interaction of biological, psychological, social, economic, political, cultural, ethical, legal, historical, religious and spiritual factors. Sexuality is experienced and expressed in thoughts, fantasies, desires, beliefs, attitudes, values, behaviours, practices, roles and relationships.*

We will all have our own unique version of what sexuality means to us, and which of the above words apply more strongly; there is no 'normal'. We must respect every person's unique version; we are entitled to our own values and beliefs but we are not entitled to harm others because of them.

Young people's sexual experiences

When I have presented to first-year university students, most have reported they haven't received enough positive or adequate information about HSRRC to manage where they are in life.

I tell them to raise the bar of their expectations for all sexual encounters. Sexual experiences should be positive, fun and pleasurable. They might be weird, awkward and smelly but they should never be harmful, painful or regretful. This advice sometimes goes against the narrative they have been fed by the world around them in the absence of quality, evidence-based HSRRC education.

Since 1992, the Australian Research Centre in Sex, Health and Society at La Trobe University has carried out seven iterations of its national sexual health and experiences survey of young people in Australia in Years 10 to 12. The survey has consistently found that a significant percentage of young people become sexually active. The most recent survey (Power et al. 2022) found that the average age of first 'sex' (vaginal, anal or oral) was 15 years.

We will all have our own unique version of what sexuality means to us. We must respect every person's unique version; we are entitled to our own values and beliefs but we are not entitled to harm others because of them.

It listed the average ages for different sexual practices:

- viewing pornography: 13.6 years old
- deep kissing: 14.6 years old
- oral sex: 15.2 years old
- vaginal penetration: 15.3 years old
- anal penetration: 15.6 years old

The survey also found that 43 per cent of Year 10 students and 69 per cent of Year 12 students had experienced vaginal or anal intercourse. Condom use had declined in this iteration of the survey to 49 per cent at the most recent sexual encounter; past surveys ranged from 56 to 68 per cent.

Disturbingly, more than one in three (39.5 per cent) of those who had experienced sex had also experienced unwanted sex. This statistic was higher for transgender and non-binary people (55.4 per cent) and females (44 per cent) compared to males (21 per cent). The average age of the first experience of unwanted sex was 14.9.

What does this tell us? First, it means that experimenting at this age is typically expected human development and behaviour. Our kids don't suddenly become sexual beings the day they turn 18. Second, it tells us that children need HSRRC education well before they reach 14.9 years of age.

School-based HSRRC education is associated with positive outcomes. According to research, 'young people who report lessons at school as their main source of information about sex are less likely to have had unsafe sex in the past year than young people who report receiving most of their information about sex from other (non-parental) sources' (Pound et al. 2017). They also tend to be older the first time they have sex and are less likely to have had a sexually transmitted infection (STI). Women who received most of their information about sex from school-based sex education are more likely to 'report being "sexually competent" the first time they have sex' – that is, 'both partners are "equally willing", reliable contraception is used, the decision to have sex is not due to peer pressure, drunkenness or drugs, and sex occurs at the perceived "right time"'. They're also less likely to report having experienced non-volitional sex, abortion or distress about sex.

The importance of accurate and inclusive language

The language we use to describe human sexuality is so important and can significantly impact the way our message lands. Figure 1.1 (pages 16 to 17) lists some of the limiting and inaccurate terms and phrases that are commonly used, and some more accurate, expansive and inclusive alternatives.

We often see sexual intercourse described in books, curriculum resources and the media as an act in which the man puts/inserts/pushes/slides his penis into the woman's vagina. If we change that statement to the vagina *accepts* the penis this does three things:

1. It adds consent to the description.
2. It describes two people doing something equally with each other, not one person having something done to them (the latter is often what's depicted in mainstream pornography).
3. It is expansive and non-gendered if we choose to omit woman, man, she or he.

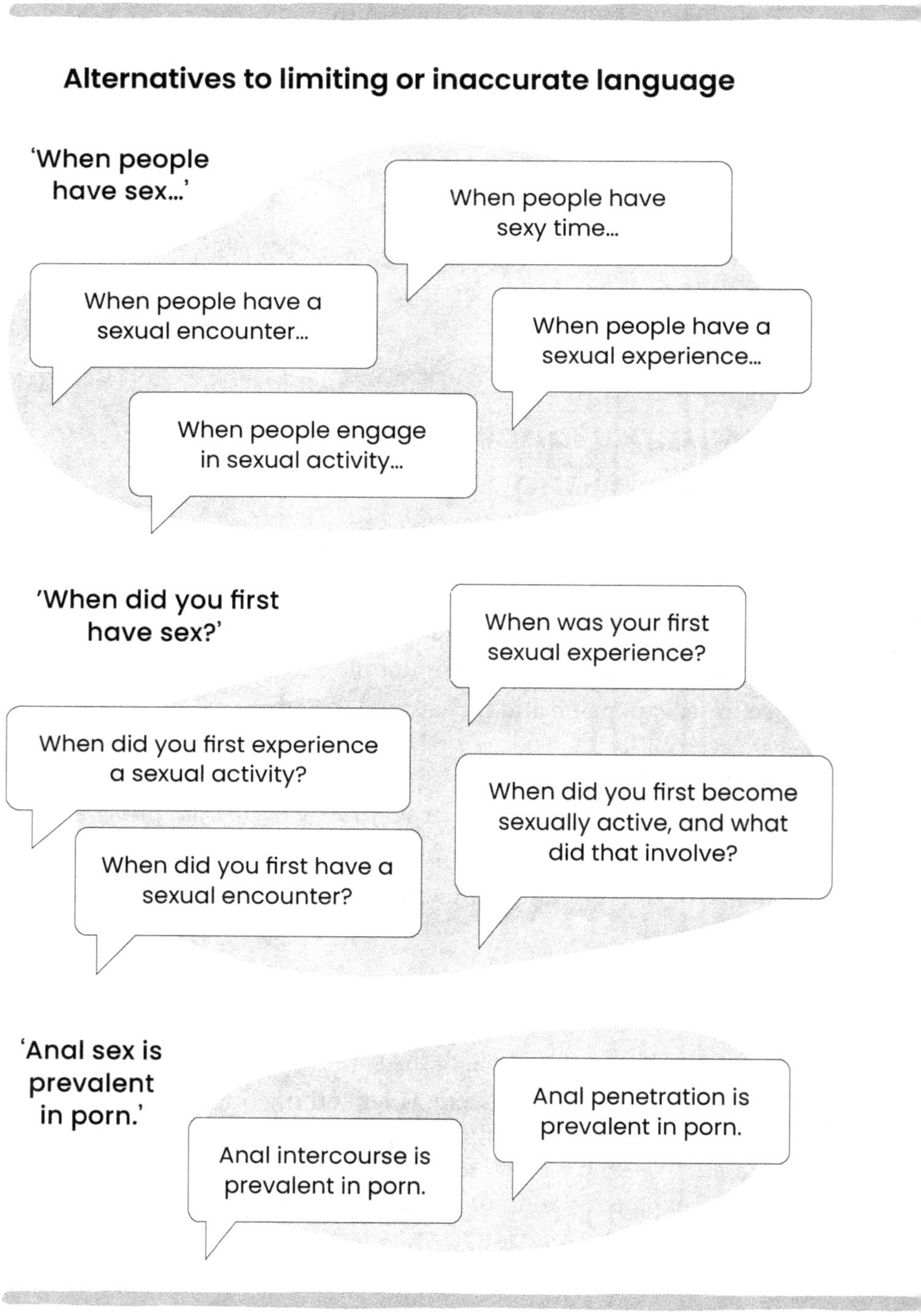

Alternatives to limiting or inaccurate language

'When people have sex...'
- When people have sexy time...
- When people have a sexual encounter...
- When people have a sexual experience...
- When people engage in sexual activity...

'When did you first have sex?'
- When was your first sexual experience?
- When did you first experience a sexual activity?
- When did you first become sexually active, and what did that involve?
- When did you first have a sexual encounter?

'Anal sex is prevalent in porn.'
- Anal penetration is prevalent in porn.
- Anal intercourse is prevalent in porn.

Figure 1.1: Alternatives to limiting or inaccurate language

The basics of sexuality education

'You need to use condoms for sex.'

> You need to use condoms for penetrative sexual activities or for sexual intercourse.

> You need to use condoms for sexual penetration with a penis or shared insertive sex toy.

'He expected to have sex with her.'

> He expected to have vaginal intercourse with her.

> He expected to have sexual intercourse with her.

> He expected to have oral intercourse with her.

'They hooked up for sex.'

> They hooked up sexually.

> They hooked up for a sexual experience/ encounter.

> They hooked up for sexy times.

TALKING SEX

Ideal human sexual function focuses on outercourse rather then intercourse

It might surprise you to learn that the two most important organs of the human body for pleasurable sexual function are the brain and skin. Focusing on connection involving the whole body via the brain and skin, rather than focusing only on the genitals, is essential to ideal human sexual function and connection.

There are endless sexual activities that experienced adults engage in. But when it comes to young people, who are novices and experimenting, it's important to focus on the key components of pleasure for sexual experiences. To this end we can refer to the concept of outercourse for the basics. I like this version based on a description by Grahame Simpson in his guidebook *You and Me: A guide to sex and sexuality after a traumatic brain injury* (Simpson 2003). Figure 1.2 shows that outercourse – sensuality and sexuality – make up 95 per cent of what it means to be sexual, with penetrative sexual activities only making up 5 per cent (if at all). There are so many pleasurable activities such as massage, kissing and genital stimulation that enhance experiences of sexual encounters. Penetration is often an important component of encounters but sexual messages from porn tell young people it is primarily what 'sex' is.

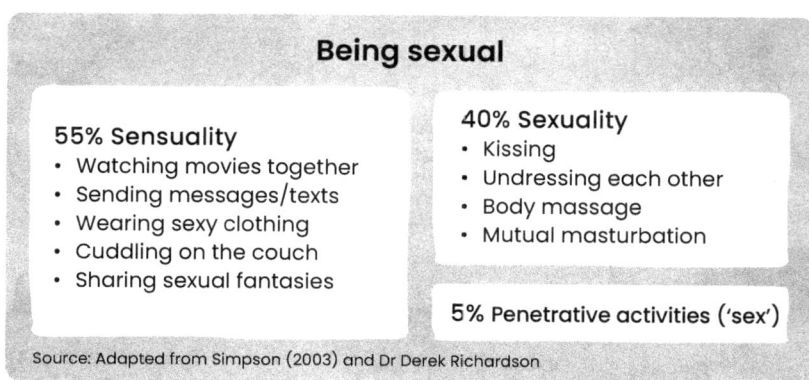

Figure 1.2: Outercourse and being sexual

Think about a young person's brain. They are novices when it comes to shared sexual encounters. If they are engaging in a sexual experience, they are learning, exploring, deciding what they do and don't want or like and trying to have a pleasurable experience. If their brain, their most important sexual organ, is affected by alcohol, drugs, fear of the other person or of getting caught, coercion, worry about body image, concern about creating a pregnancy, or worry about STIs, their potential for experiencing pleasure will be severely impacted.

Let's give them the opportunity to have all of those negative influences removed (they are all preventable) as well as to learn the necessary communication skills via lifelong education and access to resources and safe spaces.

Evidence tells us that young people in countries that provide this education well and at an early age have better health outcomes, attitudes and sexual behaviours (UNESCO 2018, Ford et al. 2021). The Netherlands is among the world leaders in sexual and reproductive health and rights. The Dutch way is to have positive attitudes and approaches towards sex and sexuality, and to start teaching about these topics at an early age (Rutgers n.d.). In a recent study, most 12 to 25-year-olds in the Netherlands said they had 'wanted and fun' first sexual experiences (Rutgers 2022).

 Conversation starters

One of the most amazing feelings humans can experience is pleasure. You know that feeling when you have an awesome warm bubble bath or someone gives you a foot massage? You feel happy, safe, relaxed and your body feels great?

When people are old enough (usually over 16), and their minds and bodies are ready for it, they can have sexual experiences with other people. They enjoy each other's bodies in a special, respectful, fun, consensual and private way that should feel awesome.

 Self-reflection

At the time of writing, the word 'pleasure' is mentioned only four times in the Australian Curriculum, all in the context of reading or using it in speech. It is not mentioned at all in Health and Physical Education or Science. Sexual anatomy education focuses just on reproductive function, yet around 50 per cent of the population has an organ in their body that has the sole function of providing pleasure (the clitoris).

Does the word 'pleasure' make you feel uncomfortable? Why might that be?

We should celebrate the clitoris and its function, but instead society hardly mentions the words 'clitoris' or 'pleasure'.

Why is comprehensive sexuality education important?

Global research by UNESCO proves the importance of comprehensive sexuality education in terms of young people's sexual health and wellbeing. UNESCO (2018) states:

> Comprehensive sexuality education (CSE) plays a central role in the preparation of young people for a safe, productive, fulfilling life in a world where HIV and AIDS, sexually transmitted infections (STIs), unintended pregnancies, gender-based violence (GBV) and gender inequality still pose serious risks to their well-being. However, despite clear and compelling evidence for the benefits of high-quality,

curriculum-based CSE, few children and young people receive preparation for their lives that empowers them to take control and make informed decisions about their sexuality and relationships freely and responsibly.

Figure 1.3 outlines the aims of sexuality education for children.

Learn
Cognitive, emotional, physical and social aspects of sexuality

Aim
Equip with knowledge, skills, attitudes and values that will empower them

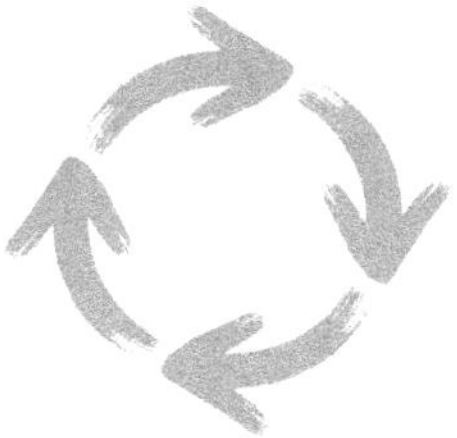

Realise
Their health, wellbeing and dignity; respectful social and sexual relationships

Consider
How their choices affect their own and others' wellbeing; understand and protect their rights

Figure 1.3: The aims of sexuality education for children

Human sexuality education must be age-appropriate, comprehensive and taught alongside respectful relationships and consent. The Government of Western Australia Department of Health suggests a teaching framework based on eight aspects of sexuality, based on the World Health Organization's guidance and outlined in figure 1.4, overleaf.

*Children don't need
'sex ed', they need
sexuality education.*

*Comprehensive sexuality
education is known to
prevent harm.*

Human sexuality education teaching framework

Safety
- privacy and bodily integrity
- protective behaviours and consent
- online safety
- abuse and violence
- help-seeking

Relationships
- families
- friendships
- romantic relationships
- intimate relationships
- respect
- parenting

Growing bodies
- anatomy
- puberty
- body diversity
- body image
- reproduction
- pregnancy

Gender
- norms and stereotypes
- social construction
- gender equality
- gender-based violence

Values, rights and culture
- human rights
- culture and values
- society, media and peer influences
- celebrating diversity
- achieving equity

Communication skills
- emotional literacy
- assertive communication
- norms and peer influence
- decision-making
- refusal and negotiation
- help-seeking
- media literacy

Sexuality and sexual behaviour
- sexuality
- sexual life cycle
- sexual behaviour
- sexual response and pleasure
- sexual consent
- sexually explicit material

Sexual and reproductive health
- safer sex and contraception
- reducing risks
- informed decision-making
- pregnancy options
- stigma and discrimination
- support

Source: Adapted from Government of Western Australia Department of Health (2023)

Figure 1.4: Human sexuality education teaching framework

A recent important Australian study (Hendriks 2023) reflects two of the common themes I have seen first-hand in my work in schools and presenting to tens of thousands of parents: parents want sexuality education to be taught in schools, and they are not having enough conversations at home.

The perception that parents are a barrier to school delivery of sexuality education is inaccurate. The very small number of parents at any given school who do complain to schools or politicians are so noticeable because they tend to communicate aggressively and share disruptive fear-based reactions, often quoting inaccurate information. Some persist with complaints even though they are able to remove their children from the lessons if they so choose.

The study found that, overwhelmingly, Australian parents support school-based relationships and sexual health education (RSE): 89.9 per cent of parents strongly agreed or agreed with the statement that RSE should be provided in schools (Hendriks 2023). Parents were asked to consider a list of 40 RSE-related topics, and there was strong support for school programs to deliver all topics.

Lead researcher Jacqui Hendriks reported to me that the study specifically sought a diverse sample, having an equal balance of males and females across all states and territories. Parents surveyed had children in both primary and secondary schools, enrolled in all sectors. All religious affiliations were also represented.

While parents in the study expressed that they were comfortable having discussions about RSE with their children, unfortunately the frequency of such discussions was low. Parents stated that they were either comfortable (47.3 per cent) or very comfortable (21.9 per cent) to have discussions with their children about relationships and sexual health. This was closely followed by neutral (neither agree nor disagree) responses of 19.7 per cent. Women were significantly more likely to be very comfortable discussing these topics with their children than men.

In the previous 12 months, most parents (72.5 per cent) reported at least one conversation with their children about relationships and sexual health. However, the frequency of such discussions was quite low. Few parents (14 per cent) reported frequent conversations. For most parents, these conversations occurred a few times throughout the year (29.4 per cent) or once or twice (23.1 per cent). Women are statistically more likely than men to report they have conversations very often or often, and men are more likely than women to not have conversations.

Dispelling the myths and fears

When I speak to parents and teachers about sexuality education and conversations there are many myths and fears that they raise, time and time again. It's understandable that these fears arise given the societal norms and expectations parents have been raised to believe. However, these myths can get in the way of parents having important conversations with their children about sexuality and schools being free to deliver adequate content, so it's important to challenge them. What follows are some of the most common myths and inaccurate fears I hear.

Teaching kids about sexuality will destroy their innocence

This is one of the most problematic myths. It implies that human sexuality, and learning about it, is dirty, bad, shameful, harmful or wrong. This is not the case.

*Children actually **will** lose their innocence if something happens to them that they don't want to happen, or didn't know about.*

As we've touched on already in this book, providing children with a comprehensive, adequate, age-appropriate human sexuality education from a young age and throughout life has many proven benefits. It actually empowers them, protects them from abuse and gives them a vocabulary to talk to an adult if something is wrong.

I'll get it wrong; I don't have the language to explain it

Your children are receiving messages every day from the world around them. Your words, however imperfect, are better than what they may hear on social media or in the schoolyard! The benefits of having conversations with your children about sexuality far outweigh your discomfort. Remember you usually won't tell them too much: it will just go over their head if they are not ready for it. It is better to ensure that what they hear is from you before anyone else, so let that be your guide as to what to say when.

They might ask me about my own past, history and experiences

It's okay not to share your personal history. It's actually a good example of teaching about privacy: 'I'll teach you what is useful for your learning, but I wont be sharing all of my personal information.'

Talking about sexuality will give them ideas — they might go out and experiment

The opposite is true. Research shows that sexuality education delays the age of children's first experience of sexual intercourse. It also increases the use of contraception (resulting in fewer unintended pregnancies) and increases the use of condoms (resulting in fewer STIs) (D Ramírez-Villalobos 2021). Table 1.1 shows the difference in the teenage birth rate in countries with compulsory comprehensive sexuality education (the Netherlands and Sweden) compared with Australia and the United States.

Also remember that **giving information is not giving permission**, especially when you add your family values and expectations to the conversation.

Table 1.1: Comparison of adolescent birth rates in countries that do and do not have compulsory sexuality education in place

Country	Adolescent fertility rate (births per 1000 women aged 15–19)
The Netherlands	2.6
Sweden	3.3
Australia	8.1
United States	15.8

Source: World Bank n.d.

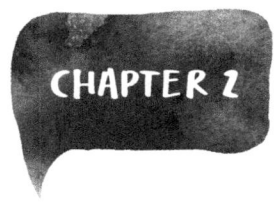

Conversations, ages and stages

Kids' questions, comments and actions related to sexual topics commonly evoke feelings of fear, judgement, worry, concern and danger in adults. Many of us learned that it is not safe or okay for children to talk about sexuality, mainly due to the silence around it but also the disapproval, limited information and formality and sternness when it was addressed. This is often why our response is to react with anger, shock, embarrassment, surprise or fumbling when our kids ask questions. Acknowledging childhood sexuality, behaviour and development exists, means we can respond positively when it comes up or when they are curious.

Your reaction to their comments and questions means more than any words that come out of your mouth. Your tone, voice and facial expressions when you respond are teaching your child how to think and feel about sexuality.

It's important to prepare yourself to be able to *respond* rather than *react*.

By responding without anger, shock or disapproval, you teach your child that their curiosity, questions and typically expected need for knowledge is just a normal part of life.

I like to teach adults that, rather than reacting with a pink, angry or embarrassed face, we should respond by thinking PINK:

- Pause
- Inhale
- Next to them
- Kindest words.

Pause

With an approachable or neutral look on your face – even a smile showing that you expect questions like this – pause for a moment.

Inhale

Take a breath and slowly let it out. This helps you to remain calm and also helps you to pause.

Be next to them

Avoid standing over the child when you respond. Sit down next to the child at their level. If you're in the car, turn down the music. Engage and pay attention.

Use kindest words

Think of the kindest, most positive thing you can say first. Here are some ideas:

- I love that you ask me such interesting questions. Let me think about my answer for a few minutes.
- That's a great question. What do you know about that already? How did you learn about that? What made you think of that?

- That is a really interesting question, it deserves a well-thought-out answer. I would like to think about the best way to explain it. Can I finish cooking dinner and get back to you at bed time?
- I can understand why you might think that. I've been planning to talk to you about what I saw when I did my regular check of your phone. We need to talk about algorithms. Have you heard that term before?
- I have been looking forward to having these chats with you. No-one ever spoke to me about this. I wish they had.
- Okay, that's an interesting situation. Let's see what this is all about.
- Oh! I'm glad I saw that on your screen. I can help you understand it.
- Oh wow, that is interesting! It's a bit unexpected. Let's talk about it.
- That must have been hard to say. I'm so pleased that you tell me important and personal things.
- I can understand why you looked that up on your device. Let me explain something to you about the internet.
- Okay, I can answer that, but bear with me while I find the best words to explain it to you. I'm a bit shy and embarrassed because no-one ever spoke to me about these things, and I don't want that to be the case for you.
- I'm here to help you. Thanks for your honesty. Let's get through it together, even if it is a bit uncomfortable for both of us.
- Even though this is awkward and challenging for us, it is so very important. Let's have a few conversations about it.

If you worry your kids will talk to their peers about the open and accurate conversations you have at home, you can remind them that it isn't their job to teach this information to other kids – that it's those kids' parents' job. Say something like, 'You can ask us anything, but not all families have the open chats that we have ... so this is not a conversation you should have with other kids at school.'

Ages and stages

Humans are sexual beings from birth until death. Sexuality education is lifelong and information is required at all ages and stages.

Adults often ask me what they should say at what age. The measure is to make sure you are the first person to tell your child about each topic. If they have older siblings, cousins or friends, that might need to be earlier than you think. When you're deciding whether or not to go ahead with explaining a particular topic, think to yourself: who will be the first person to explain this to my child? (Hopefully you.) When do I need to have that conversation to ensure that person is definitely me? This book includes conversation starters and scripts for a range of topics but I haven't separated them according to specific ages. This is because each child's maturity, interest, ability to understand, learning level, social circumstances and so on are unique and not restricted to a particular age – for example, if they have a cognitive disability.

That said, adults need to be aware of what to typically expect when it comes to childhood sexuality behaviour and development at different age ranges so that we can respond positively when it inevitably comes up in raising children.

My rules of thumb:

- Keep it simple. You generally won't give kids too much information; they will usually just tune out anything that is beyond their needs at the time.
- Always try to be positive and remain 'askable' even if you're confronted; use the PINK technique to respond rather than react.
- Keep coming back to this book to familiarise yourself with typical and expected childhood sexual development and behaviour as your kids progress through different ages and stages.

The aim of sexuality education, from preschool right through to the last year of high school, is to provide information that focuses on health and wellbeing, positivity, joy, autonomy and responsibility. It's a celebratory approach, very different to the fearmongering style many experienced in the past. Information needs to be delivered both in the classroom and at home, ideally complementing each other, with a mostly fact-based approach from school and facts, as well as values, taught at home.

In the absence of adequate, medically correct, comprehensive and age-appropriate education from school and parents, children will still receive a sexuality education every day via the world around them – but it could be an inaccurate, confusing and possibly harmful version.

When I ask adults where this generation of kids are getting most of their information, responses always include popular culture, pornography, social media, advertising, peers and the internet. Is this what we want for them? Is this what they deserve?

Typically expected development

Sexuality is a central aspect of being human, and there are typically expected behaviours and development at every age and stage of life. This starts from birth, when babies are born with sex characteristics that include sexual and reproductive anatomy. For instance, parents should ensure children learn the names of their body parts and how they work.

This section includes just some examples of what adults can expect in terms of the usual physical development, relevant behaviour, being safe, interactions with others and expressing and experiencing feelings and thoughts – all of which can be evident in a variety of ways. Many parents eagerly research what ages kids will stand, crawl and walk. I encourage you to familiarise yourself with the development that is typically expected in regards to human sexuality. The Resources section of this book includes links to a couple of great sources to start.

Being proactive, aware and able to identify and recognise what to expect at what age means adults can respond supportively and positively to facilitate healthy sexuality development, protect children from harm and abuse and foster a positive, pleasurable, empowered approach to growing up.

Children who experience atypical cognitive or physical development may have variations to the expectations listed here. Individual adaption is encouraged.

I have not covered harmful sexual behaviour, sometimes referred to as problematic sexual behaviour, in this chapter. These behaviours may cause harm to others or themselves, or increase a child's vulnerability. They also fall outside of what is developmentally appropriate or typically expected. Adults have a responsibility (in some circumstances a legal responsibility) to

Be the askable and tellable parent your kids need you to be.

To be the askable parent, you must explicitly tell kids that they are safe to come to you with any questions they have – even if they think the question might be 'rude'. Tell them they will not get into trouble. You are a safe person, and they should not feel embarrassed or afraid to ask you questions.

formally take action – to follow up via investigating, supervising, reporting and help-seeking – if they suspect harmful or problematic sexual behaviours or development. See the section on child sexual abuse in chapter 7 regarding this.

0 to 2 years

This age is crucial for setting the foundation for healthy sexuality development. Very young children rely on caregivers to gain a greater understanding of the world around them, as well as an understanding of their own bodies. Throughout these years, young children typically begin to exercise autonomy over their own body, learn some of the names of their body parts, and learn how to participate in play with others.

Typical development:

- Learning to trust caregivers – being cuddled, spoken to kindly, and cared for
- Capacity to experience pleasurable non-sexual human touch
- Start noticing differences in the people around them, including gender
- Beginning sense of autonomy, especially over their own body
- First social/play interactions with peers
- Touching own body, including genitals

Examples of behaviour:

- Explores own body, including genitals, for self-soothing – for example, during baths or nappy changes
- Experiences erections or vaginal lubrication – these are reflex responses and part of healthy development (Government of Western Australia n.d. a)

- Enjoys touch from caregivers
- Enjoys and feels comfortable being nude

Healthy sexuality conversations to have at this age:

- Name external body parts using correct words: vulva, breasts, nipples, penis, scrotum, testicles, bottom
- Positive reactions towards touching their own body (because it feels good and is not sexual)
- Potentially explain that babies come from belly/tummy/womb

2 to 5 years

Young children enjoy learning about the human body through asking questions and imitating those around them. They often misunderstand, or are not aware of, social norms in regards to privacy – for example, many enjoy nudity. It is in this age group that children commonly develop a sense of their gender identity and expression, as well as identifying both in others.

Typical development:

- Ability to identify themselves as female or male or neither, or use another term: 'I'm a girl/boy/not either' (may not match sex assigned at birth)
- In process of understanding the basic elements of human reproduction
- In process of understanding the concept of privacy in relation to nakedness
- Enters stage of curiosity about genitals of peers and adults of same and opposite biological sex

Examples of behaviour:

- Genital touching (for soothing or relaxing)
- Enjoys nudity
- Uses slang terms for bodily functions, telling stories, asking questions, repeating or copying learned conversations, songs and media
- Participation in make-believe games involving exploration and touching the bodies of familiar children in a consensual, playful, curiosity-focused, lighthearted manner (such as playing doctors and nurses)
- Using devices/internet independently, but importantly always under adult supervision

Healthy sexuality conversations to have at this age:

- Name internal and external body parts using correct words: vulva, vagina, breasts, nipples, penis, scrotum, testicles, bottom, anus, womb/uterus, ovaries
- Protective safety – body safety rules
- Privacy – the penis, vulva, bottom, breasts and mouth are private parts. Discuss who can touch their private parts and when (using the toilet, dressing, babysitter, visiting a nurse or doctor). Tell them that no adult or big kid should ask to touch their private parts
- Positive reactions towards them when they touch their own body, when they ask about sexuality or when they play games with their peers (avoid shaming)
- Reproduction: 'Babies come from ... a special place inside the pregnant person's body called the womb/uterus ...' (not just 'tummy')

- Awareness of potential negative content on the internet and what to do if they come across harmful images
- Explore types of touch and body autonomy; for example, alternative greetings to being required to hug strangers, or how to tell adults to stop tickling them
- Diversity conversations: 'Not everyone feels like a girl or a boy' and 'Families come in all shapes and sizes; some have two mums or two dads …'

5 to 8 years

Children develop a more complex understanding of human sexuality at this age through exploring and noticing their own body and developing an increased sense of self in their own gender identity and expression. Through better understanding of the world around them children will grasp the context of gender roles, norms and stereotypes, knowledge about puberty (ideally before it happens to them and their peers), human reproduction and sexual orientation/attraction.

Typical development:

- Awareness of and developing a strong sense of their gender identity, although some children's identity will not be as clear to them or those around them (adults need to acknowledge that not all children will identify their gender to match the sex that was assigned to them at birth or indeed with either of the two usually assigned)
- Basic understanding of sexual orientation (heterosexuality, same-gender attraction)
- Introduction of knowledge and social norms related to the role of sexuality in relationships

- Understands accurate terminology for sexuality-related body parts (such as vagina, penis, scrotum, clitoris and ovaries)
- Interest in how bodies work and learning about relationships: developing into an understanding of puberty and human reproduction, including one of the functions of penis-in-vagina sexual intercourse
- Some children will show early signs of puberty
- Developing sense of privacy

Examples of behaviour:

- Consensual, curiosity and exploration-based sexuality play with same and other gender peers
- Occasional genital touching; for some children at this age, this may begin to take on a pleasure-oriented rather than self-soothing component
- Use of slang words to describe body parts and sexuality
- Requesting privacy such as when showering or changing
- Comparing genital characteristics with peers
- Copying observed behaviour such as 'sexy' dancing or overheard language

Healthy sexuality conversations to have at this age:

- Demonstrate that human sexuality is positive – avoid approaching with fear and danger
- Understand that the word 'sex' can mean many things
- Know sexual activity is private and for adults' minds and bodies only
- Know intimacy should always be mutual, consensual, pleasurable and joyful

- Naming of body parts begins to include internal sexual and reproductive organs such as fallopian tubes, clitoris, urethra
- Explain that there are various ways of conceiving a baby
- Sexual intercourse example: 'When the people are ready the vagina accepts the penis, the penis delivers the sperm, and the sperm travels up to meet the egg'
- Talking about sexuality: 'It's not your job to teach the other kids at school'
- Give puberty explanations, especially in the context of the capacity for reproduction
- Explain internet use is only to happen with adult supervision – never alone in bedrooms or bathrooms
- Reinforce and expand knowledge of rights: 'Your body belongs to you'
- Reinforce and expand knowledge of responsibilities – equal relationships related to sexuality and social interactions, both real-world and online
- Gender diversity should be part of everyday positive conversation

8 to 12 years

This is a time when puberty will commonly begin for children and their peers. They will commence reproductive capacity and need to learn about it. Many changes will happen emotionally, physically and psychologically. Parents need to be flexible and supportive to children's ever-changing development and needs.

Typical development:

- Physical, psychological, emotional and social changes associated with puberty

- Awareness of rights and responsibilities related to sexuality and relationships
- Development of media literacy skills: learning to understand, interpret and evaluate sexuality messages and imagery in the media

Examples of behaviour:

- Potential intimate encounters with peers such as kissing, hugging and holding hands
- Dating (peer partners of any gender) or wanting to 'marry' a favourite pop idol
- Masturbation in private
- Potential preoccupation with sexuality; most likely trying to seek information – frequently speaking or joking about sexuality, and exhibition behaviour – think penis and testicles drawn on the classroom board or foggy bus window
- Interest in sexual references in the media
- Increasing requests for privacy
- Mobile phone and social media use to connect/communicate with peers

Healthy sexuality conversations to have at this age:

- The physical and psychological aspects of puberty
- Protect from, and prepare for pornography, and sex in the media
- Prioritise conversations about respectful relationships and appropriate social interactions; call out advertising themes – especially if it's sexualisation of women and young people
- Self-esteem and empowering self-expression

- Harm minimisation guidance for using phones, sharing images and interacting online (see the eSafety Commissioner website, listed in the References section, for advice about conversations)
- Broad and increasing conversations about sexual health, including positive benefits of avoiding intercourse – by mentioning alternatives (outercourse); foundational introduction to the importance of pleasure alongside basic introduction to contraception and STI prevention concepts
- Social skills education related to rights and responsibilities in relationships and mutually satisfying interpersonal relationships
- Teach complexities of consent and that people have sexual experiences primarily for pleasure and connection, not just penetration
- Be positive, joyful and open about human sexuality and relationships – be askable and tellable

12 to 15 years

Children need support, reassurance and facts during this important, inevitable and exciting life change. Parents need to be there for them during this huge developmental shift – especially as they are impacted by the world around them via their devices and moving to secondary school and exposure to older peers.

Typical development:

- Physical, psychological, emotional and social changes associated with puberty continue
- Awareness of rights and responsibilities related to sexuality and relationships
- Increasing independent use of media

- Increasing need for privacy
- Interest in relationships and finding out about sex and sexuality
- Awareness of and potential interest in human sexual diversity

Examples of behaviour:

- Increasing requests and demands for privacy
- Masturbation in private
- Dating (peer partners of any gender)
- Potential first consensual intimate encounters with peers of similar age and developmental ability
- Purposefully accessing information about sex and sexuality
- Interested in social media and internet, popular culture, images of sex and sexuality and literature (may access these intentionally for arousal)
- Exposure to consent and respectful relationship messages (at school and home)
- Increased use of sexual language
- Exhibitionism amongst peers as a form of fun and attention-seeking
- Unsupervised mobile phone, social media and gaming use to connect/communicate with peers

Healthy sexuality conversations to have at this age:

- Deeper understanding of the physical and psychological aspects of becoming an adult
- Encourage media literacy and conscious consumer decision-making regarding pornography and sex in the media

- Utilise everyday teachable moments to have respectful relationships conversations or to make teachable statements, for example by giving your opinion on media messages you hear with them, e.g. on commercial radio in the car

- Ask them what their peers think or are doing, and how this might affect their decision-making

- Self-esteem and empowering self-expression conversations; awareness of popular culture versus individuality

- Guidelines for sharing images online, open conversations about risks and perceived benefits. Ensure knowledge of laws and how to find information on this. Talk about online abuse especially sexual extortion (sextortion). Tell children that, even though it is common and seems fun and harmless, taking, storing and sharing these images is illegal and actually very risky. As they get older it will be their decision, so they need to know the risks, such as sharing images in which they can be identified and the associated legal risks (visit the Youth Law Australia website)

- Broad and increasing conversations about the complexity of sexual health

- Introduce decision-making about the delay of first penetrative encounters/intercourse, potential need for use of contraception, STI prevention and your family expectations/values around these topics

- Encourage thinking about rights and responsibilities in relationships, mutually satisfying interpersonal relationships and the positive aspects of mutual exploration

- Share your expectation that ongoing consent is essential for all activities, and the positive benefits compared to negative outcomes of coercion

- Be positive and approachable, and acknowledge their inquisitiveness and curiousness about their own future experiences of becoming intimately active

15 to 17 years

Curiosity and experimentation are typical developmental expectations. Learning about relationships, rights and responsibilities is crucial.

Typical development:

- Need for privacy resembling adult preferences
- Masturbation in private
- Formation of long-lasting partnerships and friendships
- Seeking visual material for interest and arousal
- Increase in sexually explicit language, conversations and discussion with peers
- Sense of sexuality developing

Examples of behaviour:

- Commencement of intimate/sexual partnerships or relationships with others
- Commencement of and exploration of sexually intimate encounters, potentially including penetrative activities (oral, anal, vaginal)
- Asserting, exploring and identifying sense of self, individual identity and orientation
- Interested in sexuality diversity and forming opinions about others

- Forming opinions about relationships, sex and sexuality based on the messages around them
- Curiosity about pleasure, shame, fear, joy and other mixed messages they receive about human sexuality

Healthy sexuality conversations to have at this age:

- Foster healthy decision-making and encourage thoughtful consideration of choices about their body
- Have positive discussions about intimacy, feelings, empathy, consent, attraction and affection
- Acknowledge that there may have been a fear, danger and shame approach to human sexuality in the past that you want to replace with joy, positivity and empowerment
- Encourage discussion about the qualities of fulfilling, healthy and happy partnerships – independence, control, consent, respect, mutual pleasure and stereotypes
- Call out popular culture and media for disrespectful messaging, especially if it's gender-based
- Encourage critical thinking about messages from advertising and media, as well as being a conscious consumer during online and offline interactions
- Role model loving, respectful relationships
- Ensure access to independent medical care and suggest contraception and STI health check-ups
- Ensure awareness of relevant laws and societal expectations around sharing images online, affirmative consent and sexual assault
- Encourage understanding that human sexuality is as unique as a fingerprint – there is no 'normal'

- Encourage an expectation of fulfilling, safe, intimate partnerships, relationships and experiences that are healthy, informed, educated, age-appropriate, respectful, consensual, positive, fun, satisfying, and above all else joyful and pleasurable

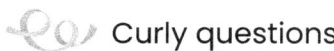 Curly questions

What is sex?

Great question! The short answer is that it's something consenting older teens and adults have the opportunity to choose and enjoy. The longer, more accurate answer is a bit more complicated.

Shared sexual activities are a physical way that older teens and adults express their feelings for each other by using their bodies, minds and hearts. They talk, touch, play, cuddle and do other activities in a private way. These activities are not for kids. Children's minds and bodies are not ready for shared sexual experiences. Children can touch their own bodies for pleasure and comfort — this becomes sexual around the time of puberty (such as developing thoughts, attraction and body reactions) then there are several years of further development before people are ready for shared sexual experiences.

'Sex' is a confusing word for many people. Most people think is a private word and not a word for kids, because it is usually used to describe something that is only for adults.

It's also confusing because it is just one simple word but often used for a couple things that are actually really complex. For example:

- 'Sex' is often the word used to explain the most common way a physical male and physical female adult make a baby. The vagina accepts the penis, so the sperm (seed) can be delivered and travel up to meet the ovum (egg). But this type of 'sex' is just one of many types of sexual activities. The accurate name for this specific experience is sexual intercourse.

- 'Sex' is also often used to describe the physical body someone has; commonly female or male but in fact 1.7 per cent of the population is intersex (Victorian Government Department of Health 2023; Intersex Human Rights Australia 2019).

How long does sex take?

Sexual experiences are different for everyone. Sexual activities stop when the people feel ready and that they want it to finish.

The specific activity of sexual intercourse generally lasts between seconds and a few minutes.

Why do people kiss each other?

Some people like to kiss each other because it feels nice. It's one way that people show that they like each other a lot.

Long kisses on the mouth are for older teenagers and adults' minds and bodies only. They are also only for romantic partners, not family.

Do people have to have sex?

No. Having intimate physical experiences with another person is always a personal choice, and everyone has their own preferences.

Holding hands, kissing, hugging or more sexual things such as oral activities or sexual intercourse are always optional. The main reason for choosing to do these is they feel good when both people want to do it.

Forcing or encouraging someone to do something they do not want to do does not make people feel good and, depending on what it is, can be illegal.

Why do people have sex?

There are many reasons (financial, force, obligation, reproduction) but mostly because they enjoy the pleasure of it. Sexual activity is for adults' minds and bodies only.

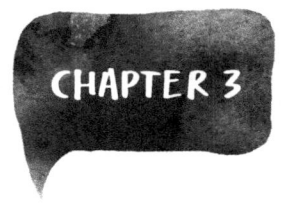

Chapter 3

Reproduction

Keeping with the theme of this book as a conversation guide, not a textbook, this chapter provides conversational information you can adapt to the many, many age-appropriate chats you'll have with children. Remember, these conversations continue all the way up to 17 years (and hopefully beyond).

Historically, 'the talk' with children was often limited to just the 'birds and the bees talk'. In this talk adults would generally tell children that 'married men and women' have intercourse to make a baby – specifically, the man 'puts/inserts' the penis into the vagina – and perhaps not much else was discussed.

This gender-normative, heteronormative and pleasure inequitable discourse is so limiting compared to the breadth and reality of human sexuality experiences. For starters it leaves out some basic facts: penis-in-vagina intercourse is mostly for pleasure, not always for conception, and people are not required to be married to do it (that is a value or belief, not a fact). Perhaps the most important missing fact is one that, if told, would help increase the pleasure of everyone who has sexual encounters that involve a vagina: as a whole, the vagina itself has insufficient nerve endings for sexual stimulation and orgasm. This lack of nerve endings makes childbirth significantly less painful than it would otherwise be (LibreTexts n.d.). Statistically if penis-in-vagina intercourse involves a cisgender heterosexual male, he will most likely orgasm, and a cisgender heterosexual female most likely will not from this activity alone (Lehmiller 2019). Yet sex is often considered finished when the male's orgasm and ejaculation occurs. The importance of vulval and clitoral stimulation (with or without vaginal penetration) for pleasure is a glaring omission in equitable pleasure education and conversations. We have being naming the whole anatomical area incorrectly as 'the vagina' – omitting the importance of the vulva and clitoris from language altogether. (We wouldn't call a penis a scrotum, would we?)

If we give them factual, medically accurate information, a child's lifetime of learning of the foundations for pleasurable, joyful, healthy, connected and communicative sexual encounters will be set when they eventually begin to engage in them. Remember, giving information is not giving permission, especially when you also add your family values and beliefs and expectations into the discussion.

 ## Self-reflection

Thinking back, it is likely you would have learned the anatomy function that a penis can ejaculate (or orgasm*) as a result of vaginal intercourse at school. But did you also learn in anatomy and physiology that the orgasm response for a vagina owner is most likely not from vaginal intercourse? Most nerve endings for sexual stimulation are in the lower third of the vagina, close to the entrance, as well as in the clitoris and vulva — areas that are not often stimulated enough by penis-in-vagina intercourse alone.

Ejaculation and orgasm are actually two separate things that usually happen at the same time for penis owners — but as I said, this is not a textbook

As Katrina Marson explains in her book *Legitimate Sexpectations*, good sexuality education in schools is a lottery (Marson 2022). I can tell you from my experience in secondary schools that sexual pleasure, specifically that of vulva owners, is missing from most anatomy and physiology lessons. In its absence, how will your child learn about this? Do you think porn is a good teacher?

The wonders of conception

The story of how we are created and born is amazing, and unique to each person. It is a wonderful early entry conversation to the complexity of sexual relationships for children and positioning yourself as the askable and tellable adult. Ensuring you are the first person to tell them about it, begin by focusing on the diversity of human experience. Each story can be quite different to others, especially as technology advances and rigid stereotypes of families dissipates. The important thing to remember is that families are made in different ways and come in all shapes and sizes.

One thing that every story has in common is that three ingredients are needed to create a baby:

- **A cell called an ovum (egg); plural ova.** Bodies with ovaries usually have eggs in those ovaries. An egg is so small that you can hardly see it; it's the size of a grain of sand or a full stop.
- **A cell called a sperm (seed).** Bodies with testicles usually create sperm within those testicles. A sperm is much smaller than an egg and you wouldn't be able to see it at all.
- **A body with a uterus (womb).** This is a very special place for the baby to grow.

To make the very beginning of a baby, the egg from one person and the sperm from another need to meet and combine. Often they meet on a journey inside a person's body; sometimes they meet by being put together outside of the body.

Sexual intercourse for conception

Sexual intercourse that makes a baby is a shared experience between an adult (or older teen) with a vagina and ovaries and an adult with a penis and testicles. Adults may choose this activity for pleasure, and they might choose it as a common way to make a baby.

When two people have decided to make a baby, they love and respect each other a lot. They choose a private place and time where they can enjoy each other's bodies. They will be hugging and kissing, usually with no clothes on. When they are ready the vagina will accept the penis, the penis will deliver the sperm and the sperm will travel up to meet the egg.

Include pleasure messages as often as you can when talking about this with children, especially older ones; for example, add in: 'the vagina will become soft, stretchy and lubricated, the penis will become hard and stick up from the body so they fit comfortably together.'

From puberty onwards, usually one egg is released from the left or right (alternating) ovary and travels down the fallopian tube once a month, often around 11 to 14 days after the last menstrual period started.

The egg usually travels for about 24 hours. If it does not meet a sperm along the way, it will dissolve. Then, around two weeks later, the lining of the uterus, which had been building up to grow a baby, will break down and, along with blood, will come out through the vagina. This is called a period. The (menstrual) cycle will then begin again.

From puberty onwards millions of sperm are produced every day. If they are not used they dissolve. If they are going to be used, they travel from the testicles into a fluid that carries them, called semen. The semen, carrying hundreds of millions of sperm cells, flows through the urethra inside the penis and out the tip of it. When this happens on purpose it is called ejaculation; sometimes it happens involuntarily, and when this happens while sleeping it is commonly known as a wet dream or nocturnal emission.

For a sperm to have a chance at meeting with an egg, the adults need to have sexual intercourse at the perfect time. If they do meet, it will be in the fallopian tube. The joined egg cell and sperm cell will turn into an embryo that will then usually make its way to the uterus.

While it is making its way there, it has already started dividing into more cells: from two into four, then into eight, then into 16 and so on. The embryo will stick to the inside wall of the uterus in the soft lining that has been building up and will usually continue to grow into a baby. The lining is special and needed to help grow the baby, so the now pregnant person usually won't have a period again until after the baby is born.

The embryo grows a placenta and an umbilical cord. The placenta feeds the baby nutrients and oxygen from the bloodstream of the pregnant person, through the umbilical cord into the baby's belly button. That is why everyone has a belly button. The baby grows for about nine months or 40 weeks in the uterus until it is ready to be born.

When the baby is ready, the pregnant body goes through lots of physical and physiological changes for around 12 to 36 hours. This is called labour. During this time, hormones help with things like pain and bonding to the baby, the uterus squeezes tightly, the cervix thins and opens and the baby comes down and out through the cervix and stretchable vagina.

Sometimes babies are born by a special operation called a caesarean; the doctor makes a small cut through the abdomen (tummy) as well as the uterus to take the baby out. It doesn't hurt the pregnant person; they don't feel it, because they are given special medicine to stop any pain.

Assisted conception

Doctors, nurses and other health professionals can use alternative processes to help families make a baby. This help is often called assisted reproductive technology (ART) (Newman, Paul and Chambers 2022). Even if people get help, it doesn't always mean that a baby will be made; but there are lots of things that can be tried and lots of babies are created this way. Some people have access to all three ingredients (ovum, sperm and uterus) to make a baby, but sometimes it can be a challenge to make this happen. Some people don't have all the three ingredients and need some assistance.

We hear the word 'donor' when people talk about donating blood or donating money. A donor is someone who gives (donates) something to another person or entity. When it comes to making a baby, a person can help make a baby by being an egg or sperm donor. Sometimes people might need the help of one donor, and sometimes two.

Depending on the family/person and the donor, the donation is collected to help the egg and sperm meet. Sometimes they will meet inside the body that has the uterus and other times they meet outside of the body, and then are put inside the uterus after combining.

Here are just some examples of how it can work:

- **Egg donor:** Sometimes families don't have the the egg, or they do but it isn't able to start making a baby. This family could get help from a person who donates their egg. The donated egg and the collected sperm are put together in a medical laboratory to make an embryo which is then put into the uterus via a medical procedure to grow.
- **Sperm donor:** People who have eggs and a uterus can make a baby with the help from a person who donates their sperm. Examples include families with one parent, without sperm, or with two parents who both have eggs and uteruses. Another example is a family that has all three ingredients, but the sperm isn't able to make a baby. Usually a doctor will help the sperm and egg meet, but self insemination is another way.
- **Surrogate:** Sometimes families have access to the egg and the sperm, but they don't have a uterus, or they do but are not able to grow a baby. A surrogate is a person with a uterus who agrees to grow and give birth to a baby for someone else. A doctor will collect the sperm and egg from the other bodies, help them meet and combine, and then put them in the surrogate's uterus. When the baby is born, they belong to the family that needed the help.
- **Egg donor and a surrogate:** People who have sperm can make a baby with the help of an egg donor and a surrogate. An example of this is a family with two parents who both have testicles. They have sperm, so they could use the sperm from one of the parents and a doctor will combine it with the donated egg from one person and then put it in the surrogate's uterus.
- **Embryo donor:** Sometimes people need help because the egg and the sperm are both not working properly. They could

get help from embryo donors. Two donors are needed: one gives their sperm and the other gives their egg. The doctor combines them and creates an embryo from the donors that is then put into the person who has the uterus.

- **In vitro fertilisation (IVF):** This is where the egg and sperm are collected from the bodies and, in a lab, they are put together to make an embryo. A doctor then puts the embryo back into the body that has the uterus so it can grow into a baby.

- **Artificial insemination (AI):** This can be done by the person who has the uterus or with help from a doctor. If it involves a doctor, they perform a process called intrauterine insemination (IUI). This is where the doctor treats the sperm with a special wash and then, using special tools, puts it directly into the body of the person who has the egg and uterus so they can meet and combine. The sperm might be from a partner or a donor.

Adoption

Another way that people decide to have a family is not to make a baby, but to adopt. This occurs when a birth family needs to give a baby or a child up for adoption to be cared for by another family. The child is not from the same biological family and sometimes may even look quite different; but they are still part of their adoptive family.

Abortion

Abortion is when a person who is pregnant needs to end the pregnancy. It is a personal health decision and can be made for a range of reasons.

Just some of these reasons may include:

- complex social, wellbeing and personal considerations, often with multiple influences such as significant relationships and financial matters
- the pregnancy compromises or threatens the health, wellbeing or life of the pregnant person or the baby.

Abortion is health care. If your child already has an understanding of consent, body parts and functions, reproduction, bodily autonomy and health and wellbeing they are better able to understand this issue.

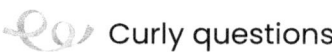 Curly questions

Why do we have a belly button?

Our belly buttons are the place where our bodies were joined to the umbilical cord when we were growing inside the uterus of [the pregnant person]. The cord was attached to the placenta, which is like a very special factory that provides food and oxygen to the baby from the pregnant body.

When we are born we breathe by ourselves from our mouth and nose and we drink milk so we don't need the umbilical cord anymore. The cord is easily cut, and the baby can't feel it being cut because the cord doesn't have any feelings/nerves. Then a few days later the end dries up and falls off.

What happens to the cord and placenta?

Some people keep them, but usually they are treated with a chemical and disposed of or put into a well-insulated medical heat box. The box is extremely warm on the inside so the cord and placenta dissolve to soft powdery dust.

How did that baby get in her tummy?

That is a great question, I have been meaning to talk to you about that. That person had a special egg, called an ovum, and when that egg met with a special seed, called a sperm, from a physical male body, a baby started to grow from it.

Reproduction

Where was the egg?

People with vaginas and vulvas ususally have special eggs that can start growing a baby. The eggs live inside the person's lower tummy area in a special little sac called an ovary. The eggs are asleep until puberty, when they start being released each month.

Where does the seed come from?

People with a penis and scrotum usually have the special seeds that are also needed to grow a baby. These live in their bodies in another special type of sac called a testicle. People with a penis start producing sperm at the time they go through puberty.

How are twins made?

In Australia, one in every 80 births are twins (Raising Children Network 2022). There are two common ways this might happen during natural conception. Sometimes the ovaries release two eggs, and two separate sperm fertilises each egg. These twins are called fraternal twins, or non-identical twins. Fraternal twins have separate placentas and umbilical cords.

Less commonly, twins occur when a fertilised egg splits within a few days of being fertilised by one sperm, which produces genetically identical twins. They will always be the same sex. Depending on when the egg splits, identical twins may form separate placentas or may share one placenta. Rarely, in addition to sharing the one placenta, they may even share the same inner sac.

Multiple births occur the same way as twins, but more eggs are released or the egg splits into more than two parts. Multiple births are more common with fertility treatments and occur in other ways.

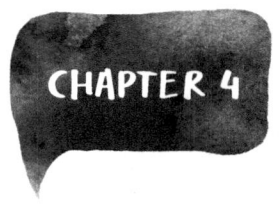

CHAPTER 4

Puberty

All adults have experienced growing from a baby. Other than when we are an infant, the fastest growth and development occurs when we transition from a child into an adolescent – a process called puberty. Approaching this massive and amazing period of growth and development should be a time of anticipation and even celebration!

You can avoid dread or fear (for yourself and kids) by using teachable moments to talk about puberty openly, honestly, positively and often, well before it happens for children or their peers.

Parents can benefit from taking some time to actively think back to their own experiences and feelings during puberty. Try to remember how the significant physical, emotional and cognitive changes played out for you. Think about the body changes you experienced, or the emotional rollercoaster of the first time you were attracted to someone. Although at times these changes are challenging, puberty should be seen as an opportunity to explore new experiences – forming relationships, discovering your own identity, increasing independence, potential reproductive capability, new sexual pleasure capacity and preparing for adulthood.

As with all the topics mentioned in this book, **my first tip in talking about puberty is to expect it.** Puberty *will* happen – are you ready for it?

It's important to start talking to your children about puberty early, well before it starts happening to them and their friends. Be proactive in researching hormones and puberty changes yourself so you are well informed, and normalise conversations around puberty in your household. Make sure all adult caregivers are on the same page in terms of how puberty is spoken about and addressed.

Above all, be positive. Bodies are amazing! If you are feeling sad, worried or concerned about the inevitable body changes your child will experience, be very careful not to transfer those negative feelings to them. Project a positive and even celebratory approach. Don't tease them about any of the changes they are experiencing; instead, be empathetic, curious, patient and supportive. Be askable and tellable.

Make sure your children are informed about all types of bodies, including the changes that can happen to any of their peers. Books are a fantastic resource to support you and your children and are available to cover all ages and stages.

Let's take a look at some scripts you could use for talking through just a couple of the many important conversations about puberty. I have specifically picked some of the more challenging, but perhaps most important, topics related to the capacity for reproduction and sexual response.

Hormones

Hormones are helpful chemicals flowing through the body. We have lots of them; they do all sorts of things such as telling us when we are hungry and when we are tired. When our unique body timing is ready, our brain will release a special hormone that starts puberty. When that hormone reaches the pituitary gland, located at the base of the brain, the gland releases two more special puberty hormones. Everybody has both types, but depending on our body parts they will go to work in different ways.

These two hormones travel through the bloodstream, heading for ovaries or testicles. When they reach ovaries, this signals the ovaries to produce hormones – one of them called oestrogen – as well as waking up and maturing the ovum (eggs) that have been there since birth.

When they reach the testicles, this will signal the testicles to create yet another hormone called testosterone, as well as start the production of sperm.

There are also other hormones involved in the continuing changes of the sexual and reproductive system as well as changes such as body shape, height, hair growth, muscle development, perspiration, social and emotional changes and many more.

Egg production and menstruation

Bodies with a uterus and ovaries are usually born with 1 to 2 million eggs in the ovaries. By the time the person reaches puberty this will have decreased to between 300,000 and 500,000 eggs. When the person starts growing into a teen and then an adult, the eggs, which have been asleep in the ovaries, start waking up. A cycle begins that lasts about four weeks. Once every 28 days or so, the body releases (usually) one egg, the most mature one, from one of the ovaries while the uterus also grows a special soft lining to get ready to support and protect the potential growth of a baby.

But if there is no sperm to meet the egg, the egg and the uterus lining that developed that month are not needed. The egg dissolves after about 24 hours of being released. Between 11 and 17 days later the lining makes its way out of the body through the vagina as a fluid that also contains blood. It normally takes a few days to a week for the fluid to leave the vagina. The amount of fluid varies but can be between two and six tablespoons. This is sometimes called menstruation or a period. Periods are usually an amazing and healthy sign that the body has the potential to make a baby. Most people with a uterus experience them. Their strong bodies experience about 450 to 500 periods in a lifetime.

Sperm production

When a person with a penis starts growing into a teen and then an adult, they will usually start producing sperm in their testicles. The body also produces a fluid called semen to carry the sperm. An average of 100 million sperm are produced every day. They are stored and mature in the epididymis, which is behind the testicle, for approximately three months. If the sperm are not used, and do not leave the body, they dissolve and are reabsorbed by the body. Sperm can leave the body via ejaculation. An ejaculation can contain anywhere from 40 million to 1.5 billion sperm in approximately one teaspoon of semen.

Wet dreams can happen to anybody

Due to the hormones that cause bodies to be ready for sexual experiences (a process of sexual maturity), puberty is a time when people can start to experience pleasurable changes in their bodies that continue into adulthood. Not all, but many teenagers of all genders start to experience wet dreams, sometimes called nocturnal emissions or sleep orgasms. It's a very personal and unique experience that is different for everyone. It is also okay to never experience them.

Wet dreams are when a person's body secretes fluid into the vagina or leaks/ejaculates semen from the penis during sleep. Sometimes people might wake up during a wet dream; other times they may remain asleep and only realise they have had one when they wake up. They are sometimes called erotic dreams when adults have them.

Not all wet dreams involve an orgasm response. Vaginal wetness or semen leakage/ejaculation is a separate event from orgasm. They often happen at the same time but not always. Just to add to the uniqueness of people's experience, people don't always have a sexual dream; it might be just the friction of rubbing on bedsheets or pyjamas that causes the body responses. Likewise, sexual or romantic dreams don't always cause these physical reactions.

Development of orgasm response

An orgasm is a really strong and intense sensation in the body that feels good and pleasurable. It can be described as a warm, tingly, relaxing yet contracting feeling in the whole body, felt intensely in the pelvic, vulva/clitoris and testicles/penis area. It's often described as the peak of sexual pleasure.

It happens to bodies that have started puberty. While children generally don't have sexual contact with others until they are older teens (when their minds and bodies are most likely beginning to be ready for the complexity and responsibility of a shared sexual encounter), they can experience orgasm on their own. Often this is caused by touching and massaging their own genitals and body; this is called masturbation. It takes practice and lots of experimenting for people to know how their own bodies can experience pleasurable touch, feelings and potentially orgasms. It is common for adults to experience orgasms.

Orgasm usually happens when people are thinking about or doing sexual things, alone or with other people. Blood flows to the genitals usually causing the clitoris or penis to become erect. When a person with a vulva and clitoris has an orgasm experience, they will commonly have increased lubrication in the vagina. When a person with a penis experiences an orgasm, they usually experience ejaculation at the same time: semen is expelled/ejaculated out of the penis. Semen is commonly called 'cum'.

Orgasm is often called 'cumming'. Language is powerful; more accurately using the spelling 'coming' is more inclusive of all peoples' orgasm experience, not just people with semen.

There is a lot of focus in pornography, and in society more broadly, on the erections, ejaculation and orgasms of males with penises. It is important to equally learn and talk about all people's pleasure experiences. Inclusive, expansive and respectful language can be as simple as thinking about the spelling of a word. **All bodies are capable of having erections.**

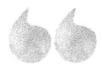 Conversation starters

- Puberty is pretty complex and interesting. What do you know already about it?
- I was shopping today and after our conversation earlier, I thought I'd buy a few products for us to look at. Have you ever heard about pads/deodorant/razors like these before?

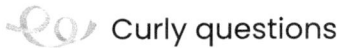 Curly questions

Why do you have hair down there?

All teenagers and adults grow hair in the genital and pubic area/around the base of the penis/around the vulva. Hair starts growing when a person starts going through puberty. Hair protects the sensitive skin in that area. It is commonly called 'pubes', which is a slang term for its actual name — pubic hair.

Why does this part of my privates give me a tingly feeling when I touch it?

That is called the clitoris. It is a part of the vulva area, and is very sensitive to touch. It can give the person really good feelings when it is touched. It is at the top of the vulva on the outside and also extends down behind it on the inside. Blood flows into it and it becomes erect like a penis does. It is an important part of intimacy/pleasure for people who have one.

What is masturbation?

Masturbation is when a person touches or massages their own genital area, breasts, nipples and body. They do this because it feels nice and pleasurable. It is done in private only. It is totally okay to masturbate but also totally okay not to. It is a good way of knowing what feels pleasurable in their body, because everyone experiences pleasure in a different way.

When someone has a partner they can communicate with their partner what feels good. Mutual masturbation is a common part of sexual intimacy for many people; telling and showing a partner how they like to experience touch is super important and pleasurable.

What is oral sex?

Sometimes, when adults are sexually intimate with each other, it might feel nice to put their mouth near or on, lick or kiss the other person's genitals/private parts/sensitive area. It is only for older teens and adults whose minds and bodies are ready for that. Kids often think that's gross — because it is not for kids — but many adults actually like it.

What is a 69?

It's an adult nickname/slang word for a type of sexual activity where two people experience oral sexual contact together at the same time.

What if the condom breaks?

Condoms actually break less commonly than people think, especially if they are used properly. It's more common for them to be used improperly than to break — for example, not using lubricant or not holding the condom on while removing the penis, or not using them before penetration begins.

If the condom breaks or is not used properly it will not protect against the risks it was intended to, such as STIs and unintended pregnancy. But there are actions people can take if this happens: talk to a trusted adult or go to a sexual health service for help — the sooner the better.

What is a vibrator/dildo?

Some adults use special devices to massage their bodies during their private/intimate/special time. These are often called sex toys and are intended for intimate/sexual pleasure. They feel nice on the sensitive skin of the private parts/genitals/bottom on the inside and the outside. Some vibrate and some don't. Often lubricant needs to be used with them.

Why do I have a stiffie?

The scientific name for 'stiffie' is 'erection'. Erections are when the penis becomes hard and sticks out from the body. Blood flows into the penis to make it hard and stiff and then flows out again to make it soft and hang down. It can happen any time and at any age to people who have a penis. In younger kids, it mostly happens if they are excited or if they touch it; this is an automatic body response. The more complex response, a sexual one, develops at around the time of puberty. When they become older kids and adults, it can happen when they have a sexy or romantic thought, or are attracted to someone, or when they rub the penis. There are no bones in the penis — sometimes people call it a 'boner' though.

Fun fact: the clitoris also becomes erect — it shares the same type of erectile tissue as the penis.

Why does it hurt if you get hit in the balls?

That area of the body has lots of nerves so that it feels good when it is touched. But also feels sensitive, even painful, when it is touched too hard. The internal parts don't have many protective layers, so it's a very sensitive and unprotected area of the body.

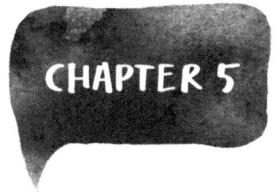

Human sexuality diversity

Every individual's version of human sexuality – including biological sex, gender identity and sexual orientation – is as unique as their thumb print. There is no 'normal' and there never has been. Empowering children with accurate, age-appropriate information gives them the opportunity to write their own script for their human sexuality identity. It means their script is less likely to be adversely impacted by other harmful external influences, such as non-factual beliefs.

For a moment, consider how you would respond if your child told you they were lesbian, gay, pansexual, bisexual, non-binary or trans. Take some time to think about this potential scenario. What comes up for you? What information might you need? How would you react or respond?

Parents often ask me how they can best support their children's potential disclosure of sexuality diversity related to their sexual orientation or gender identity. Most are concerned about how best to support their child, or are worried for their child's safety due to potential discrimination. Some (thankfully not all) parents may feel and react with shock, disbelief, fear, anger, grief or shame when their child initially discloses. You might be feeling alone in this situation, or that your world has been suddenly turned upside down. You might be doubting yourself, or full of questions.

Firstly, any parent should be proud that their child feels safe enough to talk to them about their diverse sexuality identity. Unfortunately it is not always the case that children feel they have a safe adult to disclose to. Congratulations that your child felt they could, and wanted to, talk to you. It should be a given that children are able to openly share with you what is happening; it is a parent's responsibility to create that safe environment. It takes courage to disclose something so personal. Children may find the idea of being themselves scary, threatening or confusing if they don't feel a sense of safety with their parents and carers.

Adults often assume (and even hope) that their kids are heterosexual (opposite-gender attracted, referring to only female to male) and cisgender (where their gender matches their sex presumed and assigned at birth, usually female or male). We live in a world that tends to assume everyone is, or should be, heterosexual and cisgender. Yet a 2019 Australian study found 26.5 per cent of respondents aged 15 to 18 indicated some level of attraction to the same or multiple genders (Fisher et al. 2019). Only 73.5 per cent of young people indicated they were exclusively heterosexual.

This inaccurate assumption is not a true reflection of human sexuality diversity. It is not surprising though, as most adults lack adequate human sexuality education themselves. This assumption is often fuelled by agendas from various groups in society, embedded in many powerful organisations, and perpetuated by media, advertising and popular culture.

Unfortunately, the reality is that LGBTIQA+ people experience unacceptable rates of discrimination and violence. Parents play a key role in the safety and wellbeing or their own as well as other children. You can make a difference by being informed yourself and teaching your children about respect, uniqueness, kindness, empathy and acceptance, and celebrating human diversity.

Positive and respectful language

If we are well informed, we can be prepared for, and open to, having everyday conversations about sexuality diversity. Language should be expansive and inclusive – such as referring to romantic/intimate relationships in a non-gendered way. This will pave the way for a more natural evolution for the child who is not heterosexual, and an easier conversation if it is to be had.

We'll talk more about language throughout this chapter, but to start with, it's important to note that we don't have to know, or understand, all of the language around human sexuality diversity – we just need to respect each person's unique and deeply personal version. That said, a basic understanding of contemporary language can help you create a safe, trusting relationship with your children.

LGBTIQA+ is an acronym that stands for:
- Lesbian
- Gay
- Bisexual
- Transgender
- Intersex
- Queer and/or questioning
- Asexual
- + many other identities related to sexual orientation, gender identity and expression.

TALKING SEX

Some human sexuality diversity terms

LGBTIQA+

 Queer and/or questioning

Queer
An umbrella term that may be used by people to describe their own version of sexuality identity.

Questioning
A term that might be used by people while questioning their identity or sexuality. This is common and can occur at any time throughout life.

Transgender
People whose gender identity does not align with the biological sex presumed and assigned at birth. May be used as an umbrella term.

Non-binary
Umbrella term for gender identities that may not match the sex presumed and assigned at birth or either of the binary categories of female or male.

Cisgender
People whose gender identity aligns with the biological sex presumed and assigned at birth.

Gender identity

Gender fluid
People with shifting or changing gender.

Figure 5.1: Some human sexuality diversity terms

Human sexuality diversity

Intersex
An umbrella term that refers to people who have anatomical, chromosomal and hormonal characteristics that differ from medical and conventional understandings of male and female bodies. There are at least 40 different variations that may be apparent at different life stages or may remain unknown to the individual and their medical practitioners. Some people with intersex variations are LGBTQA+, many are heterosexual and most are cisgender. (Australian Government 2022a.)

Endosex
People whose biological sex characteristics meet medical and conventional expectations or norms for typical 'female' or 'male' physical bodies.

Biological sex

Lesbian
People who identify as female and are attracted to other people who identify as female.

Bisexual
People who are attracted to people of more than one gender.

Asexual
People who do not experience sexual attraction but may experience romantic attraction.

Gay
People who identify as male and are attracted to other people who identify as male; may also be used for people who identify as female and are attracted to other people who identify as female.

Sexual orientation

Heterosexual/straight
People who are attracted to people of the opposite gender, female or male.

Demisexual
People who feel sexually attracted to other people only after they've developed a close emotional bond with them.

Pansexual
People who are attracted to people regardless of their gender identity.

73

Figure 5.1 defines some of the ever-changing common terms around human sexuality diversity, specifically outside of binary expectations. We will discuss these terms in more detail as we continue through the chapter.

The way we communicate within our community is imperative to building a society where nobody feels excluded, and where everyone experiences equality. Starting at home, we can work towards being respectful and inclusive of everyone. We can teach our kids empathy to ensure that everyone feels seen, valued and supported. Try to practise using language that is respectful, accurate and relevant to all. For example, rather than asking them, 'How many of the people in your class have a girlfriend/boyfriend?' you could say, 'How many of the people in your class have a partner?' They will hear from you that it is safe to disclose their true identity, whatever that may be.

Children should hear you speak about being LGBTIQA+ in a positive and respectful way. Think about how you will call out phrases that should be avoided and are harmful, and instead use language that celebrates diversity. We all need to prevent the appalling discrimination seen in reports such as the 2020 national survey of LGBTIQA+ people undertaken by the Australian Research Centre in Sex, Health and Society, La Trobe University. It found that, over the previous 12 months, more than one-third (36.4 per cent) of participants reported experiencing social exclusion, 32.7 per cent verbal abuse, 22.6 per cent harassment such as being spat at or offensive gestures, 10.3 per cent sexual assault and 3.4 per cent physical attack or assault with a weapon due to their sexual orientation or gender identity (Hill et al. 2021a).

As a parent, avoid slurs or defamatory terms or remarks when you're talking about the LGBTIQA+ community. Listen to the language people from the LGBTIQA+ community use, and remind your children that even people who identify in the same way have different preferences for language to describe themselves. Tell your child that it may be appropriate for them to ask someone what language they should use when talking to them or about them. People may welcome being asked rather than others making assumptions.

Queer and/or questioning

The word 'queer' may be used as an umbrella term for people in LGBTIQA+ community to describe a range of sexual orientations and gender identities. Some people may prefer to use 'queer' to describe their own version of sexuality identity if other terms do not fit.

The 'Q' in LGBTIQA+ may also represent people who are 'questioning'. Rather than being locked into a certainty, some people are still exploring or questioning their gender identity or sexual orientation. They may not wish to have particular labels applied to them yet, for a variety of reasons, but still want to acknowledge that they are not cisgender or heterosexual. It is important that everyone feels welcome and included in the acronym and community spaces.

The use of 'queer' can differ between different groups and generations. It is important to note that this word has not always been used in a positive way. In the past, the word was used as a slur, and has since been reclaimed by the LGBTIQA+ community. It is increasingly used, particularly by younger LGBTIQA+ people, in an empowering way or to describe themselves. However, some people may not feel comfortable or empowered using this term to describe themselves or their community, and may not want others to use this term to describe them or their community. Always ask if you're unsure of someone's preferences (Victorian Government 2021).

Biological or physical sex

What is one of the first questions we ask when we hear a baby has been born? 'Is it a boy or a girl?'

Humans have physical sex characteristics that they are born with and that also emerge from puberty, broadly including:

- sexual anatomy – reproductive organs, genitals, gonads
- hormonal patterns
- chromosomal patterns.

These sex characteristics usually fit conventional medical definitions or understandings for female or male bodies, but not always. 'Intersex' is an umbrella term used to describe a diverse range of innate physical variations that fall outside the typically 'expected' characteristics. 'Intersex' isn't always assigned at birth because traits may not always be obvious at birth. Variations might be discovered during puberty or when a person is trying to conceive a child and medical investigation is required – for example, a baby might be assigned female at birth because they have a vulva and appear to have a vagina, but it may not discovered until later in life that they don't have a uterus and cervix and the upper vagina may be underdeveloped.

Intersex people have many different kinds of bodies and experiences of biological diversity as well as life experiences. There is no typical physical, hormonal or chromosomal presentation of being intersex: more than 40 different variations are possible.

It is estimated that up to 1.7 per cent of live births are intersex (Victorian Government Department of Health 2023; Intersex Human Rights Australia 2019). Having intersex characteristics often results in these people experiencing stigma, discrimination and harm because of society's inclination to (inaccurately) put all humans into binary categories (National Academies of Sciences, Engineering, and Medicine 2020).

People who are not born intersex can be described as being 'endosex': their sex characteristics meet conventional definitions and understandings for typical 'female' or 'male' physical bodies. This is the majority of the population.

Gender identity

Through human history gender norms, language and expectations change dramatically and vary from community to community. Our gender identity is based on a social construct; it is not the physical 'sex' someone is presumed to be and assigned at birth. Our society has a tendency to divide behaviours and characteristics according to gender; for example, with women being expected to express feminine traits and men being expected to express masculine traits.

Our gender identity is our own personal deeply held, internal sense of self as feminine, masculine, a blend of both, neither or something else. Gender identity is our internal experience and our unique naming of our gender. People may identify as female or male (mostly aligning with their sex assigned at birth) but some don't.

Gender is often inaccurately referred to only in binary terms of either female or male. In reality, the experience of gender is actually very diverse, just as being human is diverse: each and every person has a unique gender identity.

'Cisgender' is a term used to describe someone whose gender identity does align with that presumed and assigned sex at birth, which is the majority of the population.

The World Health Organization (2023b) defines gender as:

> ... the characteristics of women, men, girls and boys that are socially constructed. This includes norms, behaviours and roles associated with being a woman, man, girl or boy, as well as relationships with each other.

Gender is also hierarchical and produces inequalities that intersect with other social and economic inequalities (World Health Organization 2023b).

Although contemporary culture likes to position gender diversity as a new phenomenon, history shows otherwise. Anthropologists have long documented cultures around the world that acknowledge more than two genders (University of California 2019).

Some people believe that everybody's gender must match their sex assigned at birth. We are all entitled to our own opinions, but we are not entitled to harm others (especially children) with our opinions.

When do we develop a gender identity?

An understanding of our gender identity comes to most of us when we are very young. According to the American Academy of Pediatrics (Rafferty 2022):

- **Around age two:** Children become conscious of the physical differences between boys and girls.
- **Before age three:** Most children can easily label themselves as either a boy or a girl.
- **By age four:** Most children have a stable sense of their gender identity.

This core aspect of our identity comes from within each of us. However, the words someone uses to communicate their gender identity may change over time. This is because naming our gender can be complex and evolving, and based on influences in our surroundings. Because we initially have limited language for gender, it may take a person quite some time to discover, or create, the language that best communicates their internal sense of identity.

At one of my parent sessions a parent told us their then three-year-old child who was assigned male at birth came to them and said, 'Mummy and Daddy, the boy has died, there is just a girl here.' That child has identified as a girl ever since (she was eight years old at the time of the session). A parent at another session told us they really could not name their gender until they were 30 years old.

Gender expression

Our gender expression or gender presentation is how we present our gender externally. It's the manifestation of our identity through what we wear, our behaviour and our demeanour – such as hairstyles, clothing, mannerisms and bodily features.

Society sets certain 'rules' about the expected traits of femininity and masculinity, especially how these are presented externally. Practically everything is assigned a gender. Even the humble toy car or the amazing pink tutu is gendered.

Our society, culture and family will perceive, interact with and shape our gender based on these expectations. By age three most children choose activities that are associated with their assigned gender, based on social conditioning and personal preferences. Think of children playing with dolls and trucks or being put in pink or blue clothing. The toys and clothing are for everyone, but we gender them.

When we use language to describe how we express our gender identity, it is often binary. This can be very limiting and even harmful to people's experience of their gender. Expansive thinking means viewing the world in a more gender-neutral way – rather than defaulting to exclusion, inclusion will be the norm. An example of this is a school uniform list that allows and respects everyone to express themselves by wearing any item of uniform. This would be genderless, avoiding the use of labels such as 'girls' shorts' or 'boys' shorts', instead having all items listed together so that any person can wear whatever piece of uniform they prefer. This expands to gender equity since the enforced wearing of skirts restricts age-appropriate activities such as active playing and participation in sports.

Fitting into expected binary roles might be simple for some, but expressing gender outside of the rigid expectations can be a very challenging experience for many people. Pressure to conform as well as mistreatment by others can cause much harm for those wanting to experience their individual gender expression.

Although this is slowly changing we still have very narrow, traditional, rigid, stereotypical definitions of how 'female' and 'male' are expressed. Expectations around gender expression are taught to us from the moment we are born, and communicated through every aspect of our lives, including family, culture, peers, schools, community, media, and religion. Gender roles, stereotypes and expectations are so entrenched in our culture that it's often difficult for some people to accept things any other way.

Gender identity and expression may not fall into Western society definitions. For example, Indigenous people in Australia may use other languages to describe their gender identity (Victorian Government 2022). 'Sistergirl' is a term that may be used by people in First Nations communities to describe a gender-diverse or trans person that was assigned male at birth but has a female spirit and takes on female roles within the community. 'Brotherboy' is a term that may be used by people in First Nations communities to describe a gender-diverse or trans person that was assigned female at birth but has a male spirit and takes on male roles within the community. It is important to note that these words may be used differently amongst different Indigenous communities and individuals within them. Other terms, such as 'queer and transgender people of colour (QTPOC)', are examples used to describe various gender and sexual identities and cultural diversities.

Pronouns

Pronouns are one way we refer to someone or ourselves when we do not use names. Pronouns were created based on gender; 'she/her' and 'he/him' are commonly used. However there is also a range of gender-neutral pronouns; 'they/them' is the most common. Some people use multiple pronouns (for example, 'him' and 'they') or no pronouns (people who go by name only).

Misgendering is using language that is not aligned with how a person identifies their own gender and/or body or not using the pronouns they prefer. You may not know someone's pronouns, so rather than guess or assume based on something like appearance, you can use 'they/them' as a way of avoiding misgendering. For example: 'What is player number 16's name? I have not met them before. When did they join the team?'

For some this might seem like 'new' language, but the use of the singular they/them has existed in the English language since the 17th century (BBC News 2019, Baron 2018, Cottier 2021).

You can also ask someone their pronouns if you are not sure: 'Hi, I use she/her pronouns. What pronouns do you use?'

A teacher once said to me that they were a real grammar nerd but were trying to get their head around the singular use of 'they', which is usually used as a plural pronoun. The teacher realised we say 'they/them' all the time when we are referring to an individual, so what does it matter? For example, if someone speeds past us in traffic we might say: 'How fast are they going? I hope police catch them before they crash into someone!'

 Conversation starters

- Usually people are assigned female or male at birth, but for some people this does not match how their heart or brain feels or how they feel internally about being female or male. Some people's gender identity is neither male nor female.
- A baby with male genitals, assigned male at birth, might grow up to feel internally more like a female in their heart, body and brain. She may identify as a trans female.
- All people in our society are unique. There are many variations of being human. People don't just have to be a girl or a boy, female or male, woman or man. We are respectful to everybody in our world.

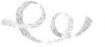 Curly questions

Why does she have two mummies?

Families come in all shapes and sizes. Lisa's family has two mummies, as you know. They all live in the same house together and Lisa's Dad lives in another house.

The important thing is that children are cared for by people who love them.

Some people have a close relationship with another person of the same gender — a woman might love another woman and a man might love another man.

Fear of gender diversity

Sometimes when I'm working with schools I encounter a very small but vocal number of adults who are focused on other people's gender identity and do not support the topic of gender – other than male and female – being included in sexuality education classes.

They often insist that people should be in a binary category of only female or male and that their gender should match their sex assigned at birth. Disturbingly they often spread misinformation, using terms such as 'gender ideology'. This can lead to harm and discrimination. Some have even tried to argue that intersex variations don't exist.

One common fear of sexuality education is that it 'teaches and encourages children to be gender diverse or to change their gender'. In reality, sexuality education focuses on children's safety. Why would we teach, or encourage, a child to become an identity that is at such high risk due to some people in our society holding homophobic and transphobic beliefs?

Safety is a human right. As the Government of Canada states, 'The human rights of all persons are universal and indivisible. Everyone should enjoy the same fundamental human rights, regardless of their sexual orientation and their gender identity and expression' (Government of Canada 2023). Sexual health education should align with this perspective and provide people with 'complete and accurate information so that everyone has the capacity to make informed decisions that directly impact their own health and wellbeing' (McKay and Bissell 2020).

Gender identity is part of the Australian Curriculum to include the gender-diverse children whose human right it is to see themselves reflected in education about being human. I have literally interacted with hundreds of thousands of people both in one-on-one consultations and in group settings. In my everyday working experience (in classrooms) I encounter children who are gender diverse. In my everyday working experience I encounter people just being human.

Some adults question evidence-based, best-practice sexuality education delivery that is proven to enhance children's safety and wellbeing. Instead they engage in misinformation, often delivered to them via an algorithm on social media. Their perception of risk is greater than the actual risk. Often not realising they are causing harm to others based on 'beliefs' that do not reflect the diversity of human sexuality, they put unnecessary pressure on sexuality education delivery. This can result in child abuse prevention and other essential education, such as puberty preparation, being hindered.

In my experience, these parents write emails to the school but commonly don't attend the parent information session.

Schools do an amazing job focusing on those who support children's safety and acknowledge and support the inclusion of diversity in education. A recent Australian survey of parents reported that teaching about sexual orientation was supported by 89 per cent of all respondents (Hendriks et al. 2023).

This topic provides an opportunity for expansive thinking. Humans are unique and diverse; we always have been and always will be. This is a teachable opportunity about respect and empathy towards everyone. We should teach children that just because someone is in a minority group (in numbers), that is not an abnormality, or an anomaly. We should treat everyone equally.

People's uniqueness and diversity should be celebrated and respected. Just because some might not be the same as 'most' others, it's no excuse for disrespect or discrimination. Indeed it is an opportunity to lean in, to learn and to display understanding, compassion and humanity. Hopefully we will one day arrive at a default position of acceptance and humanity for all.

 Self-reflection

- How do you want your children to feel and react towards others (and potentially themselves) in regard to the diversity and uniqueness of being human?
- What have you been told your whole life about the meaning of human sexuality diversity? What do you believe, and does that belief fit with the reality of being a diverse human?

Sexual orientation

A person can feel romantic, spiritual and/or sexual attraction to people of the same gender, a gender that isn't their own, multiple genders or none. Sexual orientation describes a person's sense of identity based on those attractions. Descriptive language is constantly changing, but the three more common categories of sexual orientation include:

- Gay, lesbian (attracted to people of the same gender)
- Bisexual (attracted to people of more than one gender)
- Heterosexual, straight (attracted to people of the opposite gender, female or male).

Many more variations of sexual orientation exist, including:

- Pansexual (attracted to people regardless of their gender identity)
- Asexual (does not experience sexual attraction, but may experience romantic attraction)

- Demisexual (feeling sexually attracted to someone only after they've developed a close emotional bond with them).

There are many different ways for people to describe their sexual and romantic attraction. People can choose to use these words to describe themselves, or they don't have to use labels at all. The labels that they might use for themselves are also not permanent. Each person will also have their own interpretation of these labels and that may differ from person to person – for example, people who are bisexual may define their bisexuality as attraction to males and females, or attraction to females and non-binary people. People can change their labels as they learn more about themselves and figure out what description best fits how they feel. It really is no-one else's business after all.

When does sexual attraction begin?

Before puberty, it is possible for the following to occur:

- Romantic attractions or crushes – children may say they have 'girlfriends', 'boyfriends' or 'partners' in their class or be 'in love' with their favourite idol or singer.

- Role-playing – for example, saying that they are 'going to marry' their best friend.

- Self-stimulation (sometimes to arousal) – even very young children may self-stimulate. They enjoy touch, including of the genitals, and this is typically expected behaviour. If arousal (i.e. an erect penis) does occur it is important to acknowledge this type of genital arousal is via a nerve pathway directly to and from the genitals to an area in the lower back/spinal cord (called a reflex arc). It is purely an automatic response, and not usually a response involving brain messages or thoughts that indicate desire or intent.

Around the time of or after puberty, sexual attraction evolves in most (not all) people as a combination of:

- emotional attraction
- physiological arousal (brain and/or skin)
- the desire and intent to have physical, sexual contact with another person.

This will potentially result in relationships and sexual behaviours influenced strongly by society, culture, demography and socioeconomic status.

If you think back, you may recall that your first sexual attraction (that is, an attraction that felt similar to your experiences of adult sexual attraction) occurred at, or after, puberty – during adolescence. The age of first sexual attraction will be different for everyone, as the very definition of adolescence is variable, as is the range of behaviours that people engage in. Regardless of their sexual orientation, a person's age and maturity influences these developmental experiences.

Heterosexual, same-gender-attracted and bisexual children probably realise their sexual orientation at around the same ages. However, heterosexual orientation is more normalised and expected, so other sexual orientations may take longer for a child to identify and express. Most same-gender-attracted adult participants in a reliable research study said it was during childhood that they recalled realising they were not attracted to people of the opposite gender (Hillier L et al. 2010).

I was once asked the following question by a school principal: 'You say that sexual activity is not for younger children, and younger children do not experience sexual desire or intent, so how can they have known they were same-gender-attracted when they were in primary school?'

Essentially the answer is the same as the question: they know the same way and at the same time that heterosexual children know they are 'straight'. When children have a crush or romantic attraction, they might come to realise the popular culture singer or the peer they say they want to 'marry' is the same gender as them. Sexual attraction – desire, arousal, fantasies and intent – develops with puberty, regardless of sexual orientation.

Creating safe spaces for children to ask questions about diversity

Being the main source of information for your child on these topics, as well as the most reliable source of information, means creating safe spaces for your kids to ask questions.

Before having these conversations with children, make sure you've already spent time on self-reflection and learning. Commit to continuing to learn about human diversity, in particular LGBTIQA+ people and communities. Purposefully consume media and content with positive and plentiful LGBTIQA+ representation and voices.

 Self-reflection

Are you the approachable, tellable and askable parent your kids need you to be? Check in with yourself. Do you subconsciously give your kids the message that you don't want to be asked?

Your own knowledge, behaviour and attitudes will directly impact what you say to your child, so be aware of what they might pick up from observing you. If they witness you being active in your allyship for diversity and see that you care about these topics, you will show them that you are a safe person to have a conversation with about this topic – especially if they are LGBTIQA+ themselves. Remember your kids may not be cisgender or heterosexual.

This is also a good time to reflect on your personal values and check in that they reflect respect for everyone – even if something differs from your beliefs. After all, you will be wanting to teach your child to respect others and that they are safe if they or their friends are LGBTIQA+.

Keep it simple

Being human is complex. We don't always have to understand everything about another person, but we do always have to respect them. Here are some tips for having conversations about diversity with your kids:

- Conversations about LGBTIQA+ diversity or rights don't have to be big, heavy conversations.
- Talk about these topics often; this normalises them.
- Each chat doesn't have to be a history lesson. Just provide simple information to address what has come up or answer the questions your kids are asking.
- Many small conversations are better than one big one.
- Be lighthearted and inquisitive. Avoid being being unnecessarily serious or intense as a result of your fears or concerns.
- Use books about rainbow families to help frame these conversations. These books will include language you can use yourself with children and are designed to show kids examples of experiences they will encounter in their lives and scenarios they can relate to.

- Use examples of people that they know such as their peers, family members or celebrities such as TV personalities.

- Use an example that you know your child will be interested in. For example, if your child loves a particular sport you could talk about a player that identifies within the LGBTIQA+ community.

Lastly, don't avoid teaching them about the challenges of LGBTIQA+ rights or the struggles and discrimination queer people experience around the world today. It's important to keep it factual. While kids are still young, you don't have to go too in-depth; it can be as simple as, 'In this country and across the world, people don't always treat those in the LGBTIQA+ community with the respect they deserve.' You can build up to those more difficult topics as they get older and scaffold them age appropriately over many ongoing conversations. It's important that young people know that people in the LGBTIQA+ community have had to fight for their rights and, appallingly, that the community still needs to fight today. Talking about diversity positively is important, but we should not hide that the LGBTIQA+ community are still discriminated against. Teaching empathy and respect is one of your most important roles.

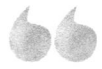 Conversation starters

- The next round in AFL football is Pride Round. Do you know what Pride Round celebrates?

- We should look through your clothes to see if you have something to wear for Wear It Purple Day. Do you know what Wear It Purple Day is? (If they don't do Wear It Purple Day at school, ask them to help you find something to wear to work on Wear It Purple Day.)

- Do you know anyone in the LGBTIQA+ community?

Human sexuality diversity

- Is your school a safe place for people who are LGBTIQA+?
- New research says being same-gender-attracted is more common than previously thought. What do you think?
- That event would not have been allowed to happen when I went to school. I'm glad we are acknowledging that we are all unique and celebrating differences.

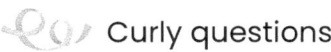 Curly questions

How do gay people have sex?

This question provides a perfect opportunity to talk about pleasurable intimate encounters that don't focus on penetrative activities. It's your chance to dispel the concept that sex is only when a penis is 'inserted into' something, especially a vagina.

For younger kids:

- It doesn't matter what body parts people have. Adults can experience special, pleasurable feelings from consensual kissing, hugging and massaging.
- Adults use their hands and mouths to enjoy each others' bodies and to show love and respect — regardless of what private parts/genitals they have.

For older kids:

- The most important parts of the body for sexual pleasure are the brain and skin.
- The brain feels and receives messages of being safe and respected and appreciates and enjoys the experience.
- The body feels touch in a nurtured, caring, kind and pleasurable way.
- Adults with all body types may choose to use their mouths on and around genitals as a form of showing love and pleasure.
- Adults may choose to accept a penis or sex toy/massager into their vagina or anus for a shared sexual pleasurable experience. It is up to each individual to choose the activity they want to experience.

For oldest kids:
- Sex toys can be called dildos or vibrators.
- Lubricant is recommended for vaginal-insertive sexual activities.
- Lubricant is always needed for any use of toys and or any anal-insertive activities, for both pleasure and protection of skin.
- Condoms are needed for vaginal and anal sexual intercourse to help prevent STIs, and are also recommended for penis/oral sex.

What to do if your child tells you they are not cisgender or heterosexual

Being open and comfortable just being themselves with family is an important part of an LGBTIQA+ young person's healthy development, and in the long term can reduce the stress associated with worrying about future rejection.

The most important thing to do if your child comes out to you is to respond positively. The key is to provide love, support and information. Ask if you can give them a hug or another loving gesture and say, 'Thanks for telling me.' Tell them you are proud of everything about who they are, and that you're proud of them for sharing this with you. Offer support. Say, 'What do you need from me? I'm here to support you. What can I do for you? How can I help you?'

Take your time

You have an opportunity to be closer to your child and have a more trusting and loving relationship than ever. However, it may take time for you to process what this means for you and for them.

When you are ready, do some reading, talk to others in your situation or get some other support.

If you have to, say to your child, 'I don't feel prepared enough to help you the best I can, so I am going to go and do some learning. Can we have breakfast together in the morning and talk again?'

Keep in mind that, for the person having to 'come out' so they can just be who they are, this can be a scary and sometimes risky experience. They may be fearful of how you and other people will respond. They will be hoping for a positive response from you. Regardless of what your reaction is, it will have an impact on them.

Make a plan for talking about your child's sexuality in the future

Ask your child how they would like the next steps to look like. Don't ignore their sharing of this with you and then never speak of it again, but also be careful not to talk about it more than what your child is comfortable with. Acknowledge the topic when it comes up in the media or at school, and check in before family events to see how your child would like to handle things. It is important to respect their confidentiality and trust them to set the pace when it comes to telling others. Educate your family, but let the child take the lead on how they are told.

Keeping your child safe

Unfortunately it's not always a safe world for the LGBTIQA+ community and you need to try to keep your child safe. Let them know there are people who choose to cause harm based on their own fears, ignorance and arrogance. Some harm is silent, such as mean looks; other harm can include hurtful words or even physical harm.

LGBTIQA+ young people face heightened risks of numerous mental and physical health dangers including depression, suicidality, substance abuse, psychological distress, low self-esteem, homelessness and more (Perales, Ablaza and Elkin 2022, LGBTIQA+ Health Australia 2021). This is not because they are LGBTIQA+, but because of discrimination – especially from adults towards children.

Encourage your child to tell you or another trusted adult if they sense danger. Teach them to be confident in themselves and listen to their gut – make sure they know they don't have to be polite if they feel unsafe. Help them to thrive, learn and grow stronger. Parental support is instrumental in this.

Work with your school to find resources that will support your individual child

Most importantly, let your child know they are loved and accepted. You should not have to, however remind the adults around them to do the same, time and time again. Research regarding young people who are LGBTIQA+ shows that rejecting behaviours by parents can increase risks, including contributing to far higher levels of suicidal behaviour and increased risks to wellbeing and mental health (Healthychildren.org 2022, Hill et al. 2021b).

Think about the parent you want to be and how you can help create a future where everyone is respected and equal – legally, socially and culturally.

*Everybody's version of
their own sexuality is unique
to them. We don't have to
understand all of the language
and uniqueness, but we
do have to respect human
diversity and everybody's
unique differences.*

*Let's envisage a world
where LGBTIQA+ people,
especially young people
and children, are always
safe and loved – especially
within their families.*

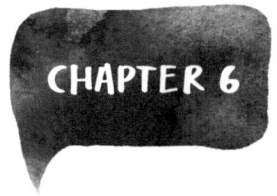

CHAPTER 6

Sexual wellbeing in the digital age

We would all agree that ensuring the health and wellbeing of children and the prevention of harm is a crucial responsibility for parents. We teach road safety, water safety and body safety, but are we keeping up with the increasing use of technology and the internet, and children's exposure to various online risks such as cyberbullying, online predators, identity theft and exposure to inappropriate content?

Children are digital natives. They have been exposed to digital technologies since birth and are the most frequent users of emerging tech. Technology is embedded in their lives and this naturally has consequences when it comes to their sexual health and wellbeing. According to the Organisation for Economic Cooperation and Development (OECD 2019):

> *Spending time online is associated with both potential risks and rewards. Children are afforded opportunities for self-expression, learning and consolidating friendships ... on the one hand, while being online also exposes children to risks such as harmful content and cyberbullying on the other.*

In my experience too many children are currently unprotected from the online world. I hear so many stories of exposure to content such as online pornography that absolutely could and should have been prevented by parents and caregivers.

I recently saw an advertisement about sextorsion, showing multiple strangers walking into a house through the wide-open door, up the stairs and into the bedroom of a teen on their laptop. The message to parents was that you wouldn't allow these people into your house, but you are potentially allowing them into your child's online world – by not teaching children how to stay safe on the internet; by not checking their online activity or not installing safety blocks and other strategies. The child in the advertisement eventually sought their parents' help when they saw something concerning on their device. Would your child come to you? Make sure you and your children are familiar with Australia's excellent eSafety Commissioner website for support.

One of the things I have always done in our house when my kids have other kids sleeping over is request all phones be put on chargers in the kitchen in the evening and left there overnight. Obviously this rule has not always been popular with the kids (especially mine and especially as they become older), but prioritising child safety is not a popularity contest. I am horrified to hear how often parents allow phones in young children's bedrooms – let alone at sleepovers.

It's natural, healthy and typically expected that young people will be interested in bodies, sexuality and relationships. Young people's sexual practices increasingly include incorporating rapidly evolving digital technologies as part of their social connections. Digital sexual activity has similar levels of complexity as physical in-person experiences including such things as laws, emotions, feelings, pleasure and potential harm. Many digital practices such as sending nude images as a way of

As a parent it's your responsibility to educate your children to support their decision-making, and to ensure your kids know you will be there for them if they want to talk about anything or get into difficulty while online.

flirting are seen by many young people as an expected part of dating. We should expect that our young people may participate in these activities when they become sexually active.

However, also keep in mind that as parents we often teach kids what not to do – don't rape, disrespect, coerce, share images or watch porn. But we haven't usually given them an alternative – what to do when it comes to respectful relationships that are mutual, joyful, pleasurable, fun and awesome.

 Self-reflection

Take some time to think about your child's sexual journey throughout their adult life. What do you want for them? What do you envisage? What role will you play in guiding this outcome? Hopefully words like these come to mind: fun, safe, happy, joyful, healthy, resilient, empowered, fulfilling, respectful, informed, shared intimacy, pleasure, consensual. How will they achieve that? Will learning from porn and popular culture result in them being healthy, happy and safe?

Sexting and nudes

Sexting or sharing nudes (sexual photos, messages or moving images) is commonly seen by young people as 'normal' – a consensual, safe and often enjoyable aspect of their intimate or social relationships and interactions. A recent large Australian study of students in Years 10 to 12 reported that 86.3 per cent had received sexual messages or images and 70.6 per cent had sent sexual messages or images (Power et al. 2022). Young women and LGBTIQA+ young people were more likely to send or receive sexual images or messages than young heterosexual men.

Close to half (47.9 per cent) of the young people surveyed reported that on at least one occasion they had been sent a sexual or nude image that they had not asked for. Close to one in three (29.4 per cent) reported that they did not want to receive the image they received. Close to one in five (17.8 per cent) reported that sexual photos of them had been shared without their permission at least once; young women (20.6 per cent) and trans and non-binary young people (18.6 per cent) reported higher rates of this than young men (11.3 per cent). When asked about how they felt about receiving these images, young people were more likely to report positive emotions than negative ones. Young men were more likely than young women or trans and non-binary young people to report these positive emotions.

Young people may engage in sexting and sharing nudes as a way of connecting in romantic relationships and building self-confidence. Like with any sexual activity, they are exploring their sexuality, bodies and identities, but in a digital way. However, sexting can be associated with risk and harm such as images being shared without consent, legal implications, mental health impacts and potential connections between sexting and other risky behaviours. As with any sexual practice, young people deserve education, facts and support with decision-making skills in order to have safe, healthy, happy, legal and consensual sexual experiences.

Young people are novices when it comes to sexual experiences. They are learning and experimenting, which can naturally lead to mistakes being made, or choices that they won't make again in the future because they learned that it didn't go well or they didn't like it. But a mistake related to sexting can often have a big impact and long-lasting effects. Young people deserve to be alerted to the potential risks and consequences of sending nudes as part of their learning and decision-making processes.

As always, sexuality education around sexual activities and relationships should lead with positivity, and should focus on pleasure as well as harm minimisation. It should provide knowledge of potential harm and risks to allow for informed decision-making. A zero-tolerance approach (especially to a common practice) is likely to deter the child from speaking up when they need help. The Youth Law Australia website, listed in the Resources section at the back of this book, will help you familiarise yourself with laws around the sharing of nude images and sexualised content.

Online blackmail and sexual extortion

Online blackmail and sexual extortion (sextortion) is when a person is tricked or pressured into sending sexual content of themselves to someone else online. The recipient then threatens to on-share the victim's content to others unless their demands are met. The demands can include more images/videos, sexual favours, money, gift cards or online gaming credits (ACCCE 2022).

The ACCCE experienced a 60 per cent increase in reports of sextortion of young Australians in December 2022 (ACCCE 2023). The eSafety Commissioner received almost triple the number of sextortion reports in the first quarter of 2023 (more than 1700 reports) compared with the first quarter of 2022 (600 reports) (eSafety Commissioner 2023). There has been a significant increase in overseas offenders targeting teenagers. This is online child sexual abuse.

The ACCCE implores adults to recognise that supervision is critical at all ages. Supervising your children can help prevent them from uploading private information or images, making in-app purchases by mistake and engaging with online child sex offenders. It's important your children know that trusted adults are available if things go wrong. Importantly, avoid punishing your child (such as by removing their device or game) if they tell you they're in trouble online. Check the ACCCE website, included in the Resources section at the back of this book, for suggestions on age-appropriate supervision.

Talking about sexting with your young people

When talking with your children about sexting, nudes and online blackmail, it's important to be positive, empowering and realistic. Avoid a zero-tolerance approach, and particularly avoid blaming the victim who thought they safely shared their image but found it was on-shared without their consent.

Lead with talking about coercion, respect, empathy, consent, privacy, and trust. For example, you could say: 'It's your phone. You have the right to decide to take, store and share your photos. However, you need to know what is legal and what is not. In your decision-making know that it can be high risk, and illegal. Think carefully about the consequences of your choices – such as crime and theft, and breaches to your privacy and dignity. I know it seems like harmless fun, but these images are part of your digital footprint – they can be difficult to remove and can last forever this could potentially damage your career or relationships later in life. On the internet there no such thing as a 'delete' key for images. Let's take a look at the Youth Law Australia website together.'

Make sure your child knows they are not to blame for taking the images if they are then used in a harmful way, but they do need to make decisions about limiting the risk. For example, will they put their face or other identifiers in the image? How safe is their phone, including privacy settings and passcode?

Encourage your children to be critical consumers of technology and society's messages about image-sharing.

You can also help your young person come up with some responses to use if someone asks them to send nudes and they're not comfortable doing so. They could use humour and say, 'Yeah, sure', then send a picture of a (nude) animal, a stick person or a renaissance-era nude painting. They could say 'Yeah! Nah! No thanks!' with an emoji of a mad, sad or crazy face. Or they could simply say 'No, I don't send nudes.'

Encourage your child to tell a trusted adult if they are worried about their online safety. They can ask for the images to be deleted. You can also help them by reporting the violation to the eSafety Commissioner and visit the Take It Down website (see the links in the Resources section at the back of the book).

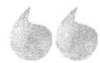 Conversation starters

- How would you feel if someone asked you to send an image and you didn't want to?
- How would you feel/what would you do if you received an unwanted nude? Let's find a quirky image you can use to send back each time.
- Do people at school send nudes mostly for fun and to flirt or to annoy/shock others?
- Among the kids at your school, is it usually the sender's idea to send the photo, or is it more often that someone persuades them to?
- Do you have any questions about things you've heard? I'm always here for you if something goes wrong.
- I think you're mature enough to talk about this now.
- I'm glad I saw this. You are not in trouble but you do need some help and advice so you might make different decisions next time.
- Does your new phone take good photos? Do you know what a digital footprint is? I'll text you a link to the Youth Law Australia website so you can be clear about what can result in criminal charges when it comes to photos.

Pornography

Every day in my work I see evidence of the effects of children's preventable access to pornography – which of course should only be accessible to people over the age of 18.

Adult viewing of pornography is considered a sexual activity by experts and the law. When children view pornography we must respond accordingly: it's a sexual activity and therefore usually not developmentally appropriate.

What is (and isn't) pornography?

Pornography is material that is *intended for sexual arousal*. Commonly it is visual, audio, printed or digital. It explicitly depicts or describes sexual activities including genitals.

Intention is important when identifying pornography. For instance, naked bodies in a family bathroom or anatomical images of genitals in an educational environment are not *intended for sexual arousal*, so these are not pornographic material. Obviously arousal may occur when viewing images of anatomical body parts – this is a normal, natural response that shouldn't be shamed. Any suggestion that learning anatomical body parts and functions is the same as viewing pornographic material is (disturbingly) sexualising a typical naked human body. It is also denying essential education that is known to keep children healthy and safe.

Humans are drawn to sexual imagery – we are wired that way. As I've said many times in this book, our brain is our most important sexual organ. For as long as human history we have shared images of naked bodies related to sexual activity; these can be seen in ancient cave drawings, oil lamps, plates and other artefacts in cultures all over the world.

It's important to have age-appropriate conversations with your children about pornography as soon as they have access to the internet.

It is not a matter of *if* but *when* your child will view mainstream online pornography in their lifetime.

It is your responsibility to prepare and protect them for the likelihood they will be exposed to it before becoming an adult.

In recent history the sharing of sexual imagery and material has become commodified via peep shows (viewing a live sex show or pornographic film through a slot or box) and in-room films; printed photographs, magazines and pin-up calendars; and films, videos and DVDs, which increased distribution. Then came the internet and smartphones. New technology revolutionised pornography, making it available to new groups of people. It's difficult for authorities to control any illegal implications such children's exposure to it, as well as production involving trafficking, exploitation or sexual abuse.

Mainstream online pornography – the type that children are predominantly exposed to and targeted by – does not usually depict reality. Yes, ethically produced pornography is available; however it usually requires a credit card and time to find it, so it isn't the type of pornography children usually come across and consume.

Consumption of ethically produced pornography by adults is an informed choice and can be beneficial and enjoyable in some circumstances. In this section we are focusing on the mainstream online pornography that children are likely to encounter. Kids have unlimited access to internet pornography on their phones in their pockets, and it is even hidden in some children's online games.

Prevalence of children's exposure

Recent research published by the Children's Commissioner of the United Kingdom (2023) reported:

- pornography consumption is widespread among children
- 10 per cent of children had seen pornography by age nine
- 27 per cent of 11-year-olds had seen pornography

- 38 per cent had stumbled across it accidentally
- most had seen it on Twitter (41 per cent), then dedicated porn sites (37 per cent), Instagram (33 per cent) and Snapchat (32 per cent)
- 79 per cent encountered violent pornography before age 18, and were more likely to see violence perpetrated against women than men
- frequent pornography viewers are more likely to engage in physically aggressive acts
- boys who first viewed pornography at age 11 or younger were significantly more likely to become frequent pornography viewers.

Australian organisation Our Watch (2020) shared a research report that identified:

- nearly half (48 per cent) of young men had seen pornography by 13
- nearly half (48 per cent) of young women had seen pornography by 15
- on average, young men first viewed pornography three years before their first sexual relationship, and young women two years before their first sexual relationship.

The report (Our Watch 2020) goes on to say that:

> ... this data suggests that there is a significant opportunity for pornography to influence young people's views and attitudes at a time in their lives when they are developing an understanding about sex and sexual relationships. Given the potentially harmful messages and representations in much pornography, this is cause for concern ...

When we consider that a teen's brain is their most important sexual organ, we need to think about the impact of 79 per cent of young people, who are novices when it comes to sexual experiences, encountering violent pornography during their childhood (Children's Commissioner 2023). Children are impacted socially, emotionally and cognitively during their typically expected ages of sexual development, exploration and experimentation by viewing this violent age-inappropriate material.

What is wrong with pornography?

The problem with pornography is not just about the nudity or images of people having sexual encounters; after all, that can be one of the most amazing, connected, vulnerable, mutual, intimate, joyful, consensual, celebrated things that people can experience.

The mainstream online pornography content that children are, often accidentally, exposed to powerfully depicts a version of sexual encounters that is harmful, and predominantly aimed at heterosexual males.

The impacts affect all genders, with many internalising and normalising an inaccurate and harmful version of what 'sex' is. According to mainstream online pornography, a sexual encounter may be based on or include:

- a lack of consent
- a lack of positive sexual communication (for example, 'Can we try a different position?' or 'Can you go slower?'); there's very little kissing or hugging
- fake bodies and positions – penis pumps and medication are used for sustained erections; positions are for pleasing camera angles, not pleasure

- power and control – someone having something done to them rather than an experience with them
- practices that in fact most women do not prefer, such as ejaculating on faces and an expectation to always be receptive of anal and rough intercourse
- strangling a person – be mindful of language here: choking is when you choke on food; non-fatal strangulation is a common feature of violence against women (Sharman, Douglas and Fitzgerald n.d.)
- gagging a person's throat with a penis
- violence (this is often met with neutral or positive responses)
- lack of condoms
- abusive language
- incest
- degradation and humiliation, especially of women and people of colour
- 'no' is coerced to 'yes'.

Mainstream online pornography also perpetuates gender stereotypes; for example, that men control women, that women are subservient to men, and that women and their bodies exist for men's pleasure.

Talking about pornography with your young people

Firstly, it's important to model respectful relationships as well as good communication.

Explain that what is depicted in pornography is not how couples really have sexual encounters. Real, intimate encounters can be so much better than what is depicted in much of pornography and the media. Giving pleasure is as awesome as receiving it, especially when it is mutual. Eroticise consent: explain that pressuring someone into something they are not into is not 'sexy': intimate encounters should always involve shared negotiation, enthusiasm and motivation.

Try to reduce your embarrassment and nervousness by stripping back (excuse the pun!) the layers of your own thoughts related to sex; your journey, fears, pleasures, regrets, behaviours and experiences are not part of the discussion. You need to give your children accurate information and simple answers to their questions. Reframe your view of sexual experiences as being dirty or negative; envisage a positive journey for your child. If you're particularly embarrassed, talk in the car – it can feel less confronting if you don't have to face each other.

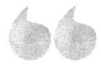 **Conversation starters**

Younger kids

- If you feel your early warning signs when you are on my phone or the iPad come and tell me. I won't take it off you, I will help you be safe. (See chapter 7 for an explanation of early warning signs.)
- Sometimes on the internet there are things that are scary or confusing. If you see something scary, turn your device over and tell an adult straight away.
- On the internet there is a lot of content that isn't very nice to see, such as about violence, war, death and cruelty to animals. There also images and videos of naked people having adult experiences. These are not realistic and could even be harmful, and they're never okay for kids to see. In fact, many adults don't

like seeing them either. It is not your fault if these adult images pop up on your screen. They are hard to unsee so it's best to try to avoid them. Turn your phone over, shut the laptop and tell us about it straight away.

- Pornography doesn't show how people really share intimacy or express their love to each other. It's often disrespectful and shows selfish, aggressive, mean, violent sexual experiences. I don't want you to think that is what sexual experiences are about.

- The people in pornography are usually actors. Pornography doesn't show what most real bodies look like. This can make people feel body conscious and impact their self-esteem. I don't want you to think that's what everyone should look like to be sexy.

- Some people like watching scary movies but many don't. Pornography is like that. Much of it can make people feel confronted or confused, or have unpleasant feelings and thoughts. You can always come to me if you want to talk through something you've seen online.

- Movies make us think that driving is about spectacular car crashes, crazy speeds and burning buses. This makes the movie exciting to watch but is not how you drive a car in real life. Porn is like that — it's unrealistic, and not really how people would or should treat each other. In real life, sexual intimacy (which is only for adults' minds and bodies, not children's) is so much more exciting, pleasurable, special and private, and makes the adults feel good.

- You might be curious to look at the images you see online, but once you see them it is hard to unsee them. Just like a scary movie they can make you feel bad for a long time after seeing them. They can have a negative impact on you, especially in relationships when you are older.

- I will never take your game or device away from you if you tell me about any images or videos that come up on your screen. You can tell us anything. You will not be in trouble.

Older kids

- What do kids at school talk about when it comes to the topic of porn?
- What experiences have kids at school had with seeing porn?
- What percentage of your friends do you think have seen porn?
- Some people your age come across porn. Is this something that's happening at your school?
- Do you think most people are fully into that stuff?
- What videos or articles have you seen that mention porn or sex?
- Do you have questions about what you've seen on the internet or heard people say?
- Have a think about the type of products you consume. Are the people in it being treated fairly? Are they being paid? Are exploitation or trafficking involved? Are there more ethical alternatives?

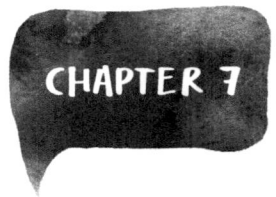

CHAPTER 7

Respect, consent and sexual violence

Our children form their beliefs from the world around them – what they hear, see and talk about, and from the stories, people and experiences that are an integral part of their childhood. As the Australian Government campaign 'Violence Against Women: Let's Stop It at the Start' says: 'Not all disrespect towards women results in violence. But all violence against women starts with disrespectful behaviour' (Australian Government 2023b). Disrespect starts with the beliefs and attitudes we develop from a young age.

Sexual violence has devastating health and wellbeing consequences. A recent Australian Government report estimated that one in five women (18 per cent) and one in 20 men (4.7 per cent) had experienced sexual assault or sexual threat since the age of 15 (Australian Government 2020).

Young people can experience sexual assault from their peers. Most sexual assault offenders recorded by police are male, known to the victim and of a similar age. Males aged 15 to 19 have the highest offender rates of any age group (Australian Government 2020).

According to Our Watch (2023):

- Violence against women is overwhelmingly perpetrated by men.
- On average one woman is killed every week by a partner or former partner.
- Women are sexually assaulted at a rate almost seven times higher than men.

A common refrain I see online is 'It's not all men.' Of course it isn't; however, we all need to criticise the sexism and violence that some men perpetrate, often multiple times and against multiple victims. Even one violent male committing sexual assault is one too many. We all need to do something about it.

There are strong predictors and patterns of behaviour common to those men who become hostile and violent towards women specifically. These are especially related to low levels of support for gender equity, and include:

- acceptance of rigid gender stereotypes and roles
- condoning violence against women
- men controlling decision-making and limiting women's independence
- having peer relationships that focus on aggression and disrespect towards women.

These are many beliefs, stereotypes, attitudes and social and cultural drivers of disrespect and violence against women. These need to be identified and challenged. As Professor Michael Flood, an internationally recognised researcher on masculinity, says: 'We need to appeal to the positive in boys and men, inviting them to hold themselves and each other to a higher standard' (Tomazin and Prytz 2021).

Violence is gendered: 95 per cent of violence experienced by people of any gender is perpetrated by men.

Source: Our Watch 2022, Diemer 2015

Feminism and toxic masculinity

'Masculinity' refers to traits or qualities that are stereotypically regarded as characteristics of men or boys or being male. It's important to note that toxic masculinity is different to masculinity, and being masculine isn't toxic.

However, some stereotypically masculine characteristics are toxic and harmful, such as dominance, violence, sexual entitlement, lack of emotional regulation and hostility towards femininity. Toxic masculinity is harmful to those who conform to and perpetrate it – it negatively impacts their relationships with other people, their emotional expression and healthy behaviours. It's also harmful to others around them, particularly women and gender-diverse people.

According to Michael Flood, those who say 'not all men' need to also take responsibility for men's violence against women, as it is a whole-of-society problem (Flood 2017). Some men will resist progressive movements due to fear of change and the shifting of privilege. When responding to resistance and backlash it's important to acknowledge that it is not about shifting privilege from men to women, but creating a more equal and safe society that benefits everyone.

Feminism is about believing in equality for all; that all genders are entitled to equal rights and opportunities. Feminist movements have played a large role throughout history to challenge patriarchal systems and to ensure women have better opportunities, such as the right to education, to vote, to work and so on.

The goal of feminism is to challenge the systemic inequalities in society to ensure everyone is treated fairly and human rights are met.

Feminism is often associated with women's rights due to the history of men having more rights and freedom than women. As a result, some people view feminism as an attack on men, but this is not the case at all. Society promotes rigid gender stereotypes that are harmful for all people, including men. Men and boys are impacted by inequality, they are taught that they need to be tough, stoic, the breadwinners of the family and so on. This is harmful messaging, and feminism is working to fight these stereotypes too.

How can you talk to children about toxic masculinity and raise them as feminists who believe in equality for all? You can:

- allow them to be emotional
- support them to healthily express emotions
- emphasise the importance of consent, empathy and respect in all kinds of relationships
- raise them to question societal expectations and avoid adherence to rigid gender stereotypes
- encourage them to engage in the prevention of men's violence against all genders.

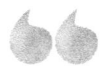 Conversation starters

I noticed you watching the news. They are talking about the terrible amount of violence in our community, and how we can all play our part to do something about it. You are old enough now to be aware of and start thinking about what you might do if you witness disrespect. Mum and I have a zero-tolerance approach to any men's violence against other people, especially women and non-binary people.

It takes some time as you grow older to gain skills and feel confident to take action. It doesn't have to be much — it can just

Respect, consent and sexual violence

be calling it out — but we all need to contribute to creating a world and a culture where people don't treat each other this way.

When you see it at school, you could decide to intervene — to be an active bystander or an upstander. All of us, but especially other males, must take action to prevent or stop a situation that could lead to violence. We need to hold those [insert engaging teen/family slang name such as idiots, wankers or tools] accountable for their actions.

This can include speaking up or calling it out when someone makes a sexist or derogatory comment, intervening when someone is being harassed or assaulted, or simply supporting the person who has been targeted or appears to need assistance (especially if we don't feel safe at the time to intervene). If you hear or see a boy or man acting in a disrespectful way to another gender, you can call this out if you feel safe to — and I'd be so proud of you for doing this! You could say something like:

- 'Nobody likes hearing that.'
- 'That's pretty offensive if you think about it.'
- 'How do you think that makes them feel?'
- 'I don't get it — what does that mean?'
- 'Yeah, I'm not sure we'd all agree with you there.'
- 'Is it just me or does everyone here think that's out of line?'
- 'Would you say that about your girlfriend/sister/mother?'
- 'How do you reckon your girlfriend/sister/mother feels when people say stuff like that to them?'

If you really don't feel comfortable speaking up, sometimes you can just give 'a look' to make it clear you don't agree with the comment. Don't laugh — just sigh, shake your head or walk away. You could also offer an act of kindness to the other person who was targeted, later. Remember to report the situation to one of the teachers at school, or I can do that for you if it would be helpful.

Virginity

Virginity is a social construct that is not based on fact. That a hymen must 'break' for virginity to be 'lost' is inaccurate. The hymen (the thin membrane at the opening of the vagina) can be almost impossible to see or feel. Hymens come in all shapes and sizes and are mostly not intact (if they ever were) by the time a person might choose to experience sexual penetration.

One traditional concept of virginity commonly refers to penis-in-vagina sex as though that is what sex is – and that it can only occur between a married man and woman. Penis-in-vagina intercourse is said to be the main way to have sex. This disregards other forms of sexual activities, as well as people whose experiences vary from heterosexuality. As Otis says on the fabulous Netflix series Sex Education (2021): 'Hand jobs are sex. Virginity is a construct.'

It also results in inequality around pleasure, prioritising the sexual pleasure of the penis owner. Most people with a vagina do not orgasm from just penetration; only 18 to 30 per cent of heterosexual women always or usually orgasm during vaginal sexual intercourse alone (Lehmiller 2019, Herbenick et al. 2018). The orgasm gap is real, regardless of which activities are involved. A recent study revealed that 95 per cent of heterosexual men usually or always orgasm when sexually intimate, compared to 65 per cent of heterosexual women (Frederick et al. 2018).

Virginity has often been equated with a woman's purity, and therefore her worth. It perpetuates rigid gender roles, and implies that women and girls should remain pure and dress modestly to prevent male counterparts from getting distracted or giving into sexual urges. There are many more patriarchal and harmful problems with the term.

The concept of virginity has been used to control women and girls for centuries.

Male virginity isn't expected to be proven.

Virginity is a way for women's sexuality to be controlled by men. It's another example of patriarchy.

Historically, and today in some cultures, it is thought a virgin will bleed due to a broken or penetrated hymen during their first penetrative vaginal sexual encounter. It is a pervasive social myth that a 'virgin' will bleed, which can lead to shame in some communities if this does not happen on her wedding night, suggesting she has had vaginal 'sex' before. In reality, people do not always experience bleeding with their first vaginal penetration regardless of what is involved (for example finger, tampon, sex toy or penis), so this expectation is usually impossible to meet. Further, the practice of virginity testing exacerbates the belief that 'sex' is mainly a penis being inserted into a vagina and that it is acceptable and even celebrated to cause physical trauma and pain. Also, the idea that the first night of marriage must equate to heterosexual penetrative sex is problematic for many reasons – too many to address here. Imagine instead that the participants are afforded privacy and free consent to choose sexual activity or not. And, if they do wish to focus on outercourse, that it involves plenty of lubricant and no requirement to cause any tissue damage or bleeding.

We should teach our kids that 'sex' means different things to different people and there are all sorts of different sexual encounters. 'Sex' doesn't just involve a man inserting his penis into a woman's vagina. Sexual encounters involve people of all sorts of gender identities, body parts and sexual preferences.

Instead of describing people as 'losing their virginity' we could describe it as 'gaining' or having a 'first-ever' experience (of orgasm, kissing, mutual masturbation and so on – choose your own adventure). It is their 'sexual debut'! This could describe when someone has their first sexual experience with another person, or each individual person could define when their own sexual debut is; it is not limited to one certain type of sexual act (that benefits the patriarchy). After all, is it really anyone else's business?

Consent

Teaching our children about consent is actually teaching them about the fundamentals of being human. Consent is integral to lifelong human relationships. We must empower children with internal decision-making skills and knowledge of the nuances of consent communication early, so that they can take those skills with them into all of their relationships throughout life – including intimate and sexual encounters when they are older. Age-appropriate consent conversations for younger children often have nothing to do with sexual encounters; however we do need to explicitly teach sexual consent to older kids.

Consent underpins all relationships, which are essential to humanity. It's about showing kindness, compassion, empathy and respect, and fostering connection, communication and safety. Consent is permission, reciprocity and generosity. It's how we show respect for ourselves and others. It's about wanting the best for ourselves and others.

To contribute to solving the epidemic of gender-based violence in Australia, consent needs to be taught from a young age (age appropriately) and be based on a positive framework, well before they are sexually active. Taught consistently, in plain language, relevant and appropriate, with a focus on breaking down rigid gender stereotypes and disrespect, we can create a positive consent culture, where children's default position is to ask: 'Is everyone safe? Am I providing a safe space for others? Do I feel safe?'

Consent is permission for shared experiences that can result in immense and (potentially) limitless happiness, joy and pleasure. Human love, both sexual and non-sexual, requires consent.

If we value consent it means that we value respect for others; that we want our relationships and human connections to be positive, healthy and most importantly pleasurable and joyful. Acting with respect and ensuring there is consent at all times prevents us from causing harm to others.

Consent can be both simple and complex

Consent can be as simple as an enthusiastic, ongoing, mutually negotiated, affirmative and enjoyable 'YES'!

But it is usually more complex, because being human is complex. In different situations, humans can experience a range of different feelings, thoughts and emotions. We need to make important choices to be sure that someone wants to share an experience equally and that they are giving affirmative permission – and that, equally, we give consent.

The basic principles of consent must always apply to all of our connections including family, friends, professional, caregiving and receiving, cultural, religious, intimate, sexual and even our connections with strangers.

Consent is about making fundamental decisions; it's not just about actions.

Consent can be verbal and nonverbal. It's about trying to understand how the other person might feel rather than just hearing their words (see figure 7.1).

Consent keeps everyone's bodies, feelings and thoughts comfortable and safe. It respects that everyone has their own personal body space, feelings and thoughts. In a healthy partnership, all people can speak freely and everyone feels positive and safe because they can communicate their expectations and what they want.

When it comes to gender-based non-consensual situations, a key factor is that women especially have been (and continue to be) conditioned to say yes and be compliant. This is due to a variety of societal and cultural factors, predominantly the patriarchal nature of many societies where men hold more

What can consent sound like? (Spoken words, tone, sounds)

- Yes
- I'm so sure
- I know
- I'm excited
- Let's keep doing th.is, it's fun!
- Woohoo! Yippee! Zip-a-dee-doodah!
- More!
- I want to
- I'm not worried
- I want you/it/that
- Can you please do …
- I still want to
- That feels good
- This is cool!
- I love this
- I want to do this right now. Can we play it this way?
- I feel good about this
- I'm ready
- YES!
- That sounds like fun, let's do it
- Absolutely!

What can non-consent sound like? (Spoken words, tone, sounds)

- No
- I'm not sure
- I don't know
- I'm scared
- Stop
- Silence
- No more
- I want to but…
- Wait, I feet worried about …
- I don't want you/it/that
- Can you please not do …
- I thought I wanted to play but …
- That hurts, please don't hug me so tightly
- Maybe
- That doesn't sound like fun
- That sounds like fun, but not right now
- Can I think about it?
- I want to play, but not right now/this way
- I don't know how I feel about this
- I'm not sure I'm ready yet
- I don't want to do this anymore
- This feels wrong

What can consent look like? (Body language)

- Thumbs up
- Nodding
- Moving towards the person
- Opening arms for a hug
- Smiling
- Making direct eye contact
- Being responsive
- Being vocal
- Looking visibly happy
- Looking relaxed

What can non-consent look like? (Body language)

- Thumbs down
- Shaking head
- Moving away
- Folding arms
- Frowning
- Not making eye contact
- Not being responsive
- Being silent
- Looking visibly upset
- Flinching away from a person/moving away

Figure 7.1: Examples of what consent and non-consent can sound and look like

power and authority than women and other genders. This power dynamic can lead to genders other than males feeling pressure to comply with men's wishes and desires to avoid conflict or negative consequences. Pornography often depicts cisgendered heterosexual scenarios where a woman gives into a man and does as he says.

Women are often socialised from a young age to prioritise the needs and wants of others over their own. This can lead to a tendency to say yes and be compliant in order to please others or avoid being seen as difficult or confrontational.

Another factor is the prevalence of gender stereotypes that portray women and non-binary people, especially, as passive, nurturing and submissive. These stereotypes can reinforce the idea that people of any gender with these traits should be compliant to society's stereotypical expectations of masculinity – such as being dominant and powerful.

Above all, consent is a human right. Sexual consent is also the law – for good reason.

The principles of consent

My previous co-author Ingrid Laguna and I compiled the following list of principles around consent that can be taught to young people in an age-appropriate way. Some of these principles are essential to obtaining and giving consent, while others enhance consent, making relationships and experiences the best they can be.

The book Ingrid and I co-authored – *Kit and Arlo Find a Way* – and the associated website are great resources to support parents and educators in teaching these concepts to eight to 12-year-olds. See the Resources section of this book for more information.

Positive consent decisions are about:

- being honest
- trusting others
- respecting others
- being ethical
- making mutual decisions
- ensuring everyone is equal
- taking responsibility that everyone is happy with what is happening
- communicating what we want and need, while paying attention to what others want and need.

Positive consent actions are about:

- valuing friendships
- enjoying playing and having fun
- awareness of how we impact others
- making sure we always act within the law
- actively giving and receiving permission
- creating a space for others to speak freely
- respecting people's human rights and bodily autonomy
- exercising mutual agreement and negotiation in all shared activities
- allowing people to withdraw consent
- always being kind and considerate to others
- never coercing, bribing or forcing someone.

Positive consent communication is:

- enthusiastic
- ongoing
- clear
- affirmative
- shared agreement
- verbal and nonverbal.

Positive consent thoughts and feelings:

- exercise genuine empathy for others
- value the comfort of others
- manage disappointment and expectations
- acknowledge personal courage in ourselves and others
- are based on respect, generosity, reciprocity, human connection and gratitude
- are rooted in responsibility for our actions.

Positive consent beliefs:

- respect diversity
- don't adhere to rigid gender stereotypes
- value that no-one has power over another person
- promote equity in all human relationships.

Let's teach our children that consent doesn't have to be awkward or weird to negotiate, and that sexual experiences feel better for everyone when consent is at the centre. But consent does involve courage – especially to withdraw it.

Talking about consent with your young person

When speaking with young people about consent I like to speak of it in a positive way. It is not sexy to have to talk someone into something – you don't actually have the other person's consent if you coerced them to say yes. It is much sexier when both people are 'into it' and want to explore and play. Everything you do together should be pleasant and enjoyable for all involved.

During sexual encounters you should not feel as though you are being pushed far out of your comfort zone. It is normal to experiment, but you don't have to go out of your comfort zone because someone else wants you to or makes you feel like you should.

When exploring a brand-new activity or experience together, even if you are unsure while navigating it, as a minimum you must have mutual, clear, ongoing agreement, motivation and enthusiasm to continue at all times. This ensures a consensual, legal and respectful encounter with the likely bonus of awesome and fun experiences with another person.

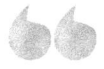 Conversation starters

- There are a few key things you have to learn before you start having relationships and dating.
- The legal age of consent for penetrative sex is 16, and there is a pretty good reason for this …
- Kissing someone without asking is not okay. Coercion is not okay, ever. If someone says no, then it is no. What do you think about this TV show promoting this?
- Actually that show is unrealistic and misleading … sexual experiences are actually awesome and pleasurable when both people are completely 'into it'.

- Negotiating a mutually enjoyable activity to do together will mean you both have the best experience. What could you say to check in that they are still keen on it?
- How would you describe people's options for feeling comfortable, private and able to be fully 'into it' if they are having a sexual encounter at a party? Do you think people are in a position to give ongoing, informed and enthusiastic agreement/consent when they are at a party and might have been drinking?
- Have you and your partner talked about what you are comfortable doing sexually? How might this change as your relationship progresses?
- Do you ever wonder if one of your friends has had a risky experience with a partner?
- It's hard to trust your own judgement/gut feelings when someone is trying to convince you to do something you're not sure about. Does that happen in your group of friends?

Child sexual abuse

Prevention of child sexual abuse (CSA) is a whole-of-society responsibility.

There are many misconceptions about CSA. Parents often focus on stranger danger, without giving enough attention to the reality that, in 86 per cent of cases (likely more due to underreporting), the CSA perpetrator is known to the victim (Australian Government 2022b). RAINN, the largest anti-sexual assault service in the US, quotes this figure at 93 per cent (RAINN n.d.). Parents need to deliver very specific education, from an early age, in line with the facts we know about CSA. There are excellent resources available to parents (see the Resources section at the back of this book to start) and I encourage you to be proactive in your research. You must educate your children in body safety and protecting themselves online, just as you give them swimming lessons and teach them about healthy living and road safety.

What is CSA?

CSA occurs when contact or non-contact non-consensual sexual acts are inflicted on a child by another person (an adult or child) (Higgins 2023). It includes many different activities such as:

- sexual touching
- oral sex or vaginal or anal penetration
- indecent exposure
- exposing children to sexual acts or pictures
- enticing children to engage in sexual internet chat and image-sharing (such as through games) (Government of Western Australia n.d. b).

The Australian Child Maltreatment Study released in April 2023 reported 'deeply sobering' statistics about the prevalence of CSA. It showed that it is 'widespread in Australia and associated with early and persistent harm'. The report states that CSA 'remains an urgent national problem' (Australian Child Maltreatment Study 2023).

The 2021 survey of 3500 16-to-24-year-olds found that:

- 25.7 per cent had been victims of CSA
- more than one in three girls (35.2 per cent) and one in seven boys (14.5 per cent) had been victims of child sexual abuse – girls experience 2.5 times the rate of CSA as boys
- one in 12 had experienced forced sex (rape)

I challenge every parent or carer to think about whether you have done as much research about child sexual abuse, particularly the prevention of it, as you did for your last big-ticket-item purchase, such as a car or an expensive household appliance.

- when a child experiences CSA it rarely happens once:
    - 78 per cent: more than one time
    - 42 per cent: more than six times
    - 11 per cent: more than 50 times (Australian Child Maltreatment Study 2023).

Alarmingly, Australian studies have found that between 30 and 60 per cent of all experiences of CSA are the result of other children and young people who have displayed or engaged in problematic and harmful sexual behaviours (Australian Government 2017, NSW Government n.d.). Such abuse often involves an older child or young person having coerced or forced a child who is younger, smaller or where there were marked developmental differences. This is strongly associated with children who are exposed to other child abuse such as neglect, trauma and family violence, have had experiences of childhood sexual abuse themselves, societal expectations related to gender norms and early exposure to pornographic material (NSW Government n.d.).

We must not minimise the harm caused to victims themselves, however we should also avoid demonising or labelling the children and young people engaging in abusive behaviour by calling them perpetrators or sex offenders. They are still developing and growing, and labelling may shame them and deter them and their families from engaging with treatment and support. If a child's sexual activity is out of the ordinary for their age, regardless of whether or not there is an apparent power imbalance, professional help should be sought (Australian Government 2018).

What is grooming?

Grooming is when a person prepares a child and their parents, carers and environment for sexual abuse. Grooming can happen in a relatively short period, but usually involves building a trusting relationship with a child or family over many weeks, months and years. This allows the person who is grooming to spend more and more time with the child. It lays the groundwork for sexual abuse later on (Raising Children Network 2023).

Every adult who cares for children should make themselves aware of the insidious crime of grooming. According to the law, grooming is when a person engages in predatory conduct to prepare a child or young person for sexual activity at a later time, and it is against the law.

At a conference in 2023 I saw the most powerful speech I have ever heard, from Grace Tame, Australian advocate for survivors of sexual assault and the 2021 Australian of the Year. In October 2021, during Child Sexual Abuse Awareness Week, Tame took to Twitter and dedicated a tweet per day to highlight the six typical phases of grooming. I highly recommend watching the video about these tweets that is listed in the Resources section of this book.

Tame implores adults to learn the six stages of grooming (Tame 2021, Jepsten 2021):

1. **Targeting:** The perpetrator identifies a vulnerable person to target. All children are vulnerable due to things such as power imbalances, but it's important to take extra care of children with added vulnerabilities such as disability or limited parent supervision.

2. **Gaining trust:** Children are lulled into a false sense of trust via seemingly harmless interactions. They're often given

special attention, presents, treats, games and one-on-one time spent with the perpetrator.

3. **Filing a need:** Perpetrators identifying a specific gap in the target's support network that they can fulfil. For example they might become a caring and reliable family friend.

4. **Isolating:** Once they have a bond with the child they drive wedges between them and their support networks. This can lessen the chance of disclosure, ensuring secrecy.

5. **Sexualising:** Sexual references are subtly and continuously infused into interactions; for example, 'innocent' touching, 'accidental' sexual contact or confusing the child's perception of appropriate behaviour.

6. **Maintaining control:** Perpetrators maintain control by 'striking a perfect balance between causing pain and providing relief from it' (Tame 2021).

Being groomed is never the target's fault. Listen to and support them, believe them, take them seriously, reassure them that they have done the right thing by telling you and help them seek support.

In terms of what grooming is (and isn't), it's also important to understand that sexuality education is not grooming. Misusing the term 'grooming' in this way is inaccurate, ill-informed, dangerous and ignorant on so many levels. Some people intentionally generate fear around these topics and therefore try to prevent education. I have witnessed this first-hand. In my opinion this only serves to facilitate perpetrators' continued grooming and abusing. Perpetrators' best weapon is silencing children, especially vulnerable children – those who are uneducated about their bodies, rights and relationships.

When adults – even politicians and policy-makers, in many jurisdictions – try to block evidence-based, age-appropriate, accurate, comprehensive sexuality education, this prevents body safety and other health and wellbeing education being delivered to children.

What you can do

Be the askable and tellable parent your child needs you to be, and help them identify other trusted adults they can go to.

Teach your children about body safety and the accurate names for body parts. Teach them which body parts (including their mouth) are 'just for them'. This gives them the vocabulary to report anything that is wrong. Introduce the ideas of 'body safety rules' and 'early warning signs' to your child (see figures 7.2 and 7.3). Educate2Empower has created free body safety resource posters, some in more than 17 languages, for parents to download (see the Resources section at the back of the book). I recommend displaying these in your home – when my children were young, we used to have the body safety rules poster on the back of the toilet door.

(Right) Figure 7.2: Body safety rules
Source: Educate2Empower (n.d.)

Respect, consent and sexual violence

My Body Safety Rules

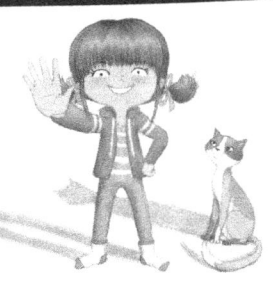

My body is my body and it belongs to me!

I can say, 'No!' if I don't want to kiss or hug someone.
I can give them a high five, shake their hand or blow them a kiss.
I am the boss of my body and what I say goes!

I have a Safety Network

These are five adults I trust. I can tell these people anything and they will believe me.

If I feel worried, scared or unsure, I can tell someone on my Safety Network how I am feeling and why I feel this way.

Early Warning Signs

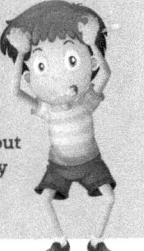

If I feel frightened or unsafe I may sweat a lot, get a sick tummy, become shaky and my heart might beat really fast.

These feelings are called my Early Warning Signs. If I feel this way about anything, I must tell an adult on my Safety Network straightaway.

Secrets

I should never keep secrets that make me feel bad or uncomfortable. If someone asks me to keep a secret that makes me feel bad or unsafe, I must tell an adult on my Safety Network straightaway!

Private Parts

My private parts are the parts of my body under my bathing suit. (My mouth is a private part too.) I always call my private parts by their correct names. No one can touch my private parts. No one can ask me to touch their private parts. And no one should show me pictures of private parts. If any of these things happen, I must tell a trusted adult on my Safety Network straightaway.

© UpLoad Publishing Pty Ltd
For more information go to **www.e2epublishing.info**

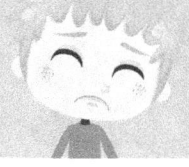
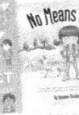
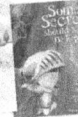
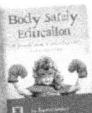

TALKING SEX

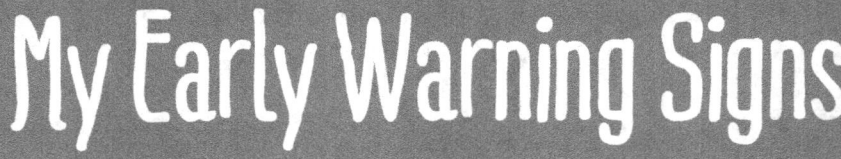

My Early Warning Signs

If I feel <u>unsafe</u> my body lets me know.

Here is how!

- Hair feels like it is standing on end
- Sweaty brow
- Start to cry
- Heart beats fast
- Goosebumps
- Feel sick in the tummy
- Sweaty palms
- Need to go to the toilet
- Shaky all over
- Wobbly legs

If I feel unsafe, I must tell a trusted adult on my <u>Safety Network</u> straightaway!

© UpLoad Publishing Pty Ltd
For more information go to **www.e2epublishing.info**

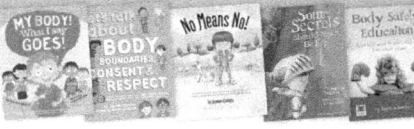

It's best to avoid using the terms 'good touch' and 'bad touch' when talking to children about sexual abuse prevention – these words can be confusing and misleading to children. It is important to instead use very clear and specific language to describe appropriate/safe and inappropriate/unsafe touching. Parents and caregivers can teach children that their private parts are their own and that no-one should touch them without their permission – except when it comes to their health and safety.

When they were little, one of my children once had an old dirty bandage hanging off their leg. They were running away from me as I was trying to get close to take it off. They stopped with hand held out and said 'Stop! This is my body I say what goes!' So I did. They took the bandage off themselves. I was very proud that my body safety education had worked – however, it was a good reminder to reinforce that kids don't always get to make decisions about their bodies when it comes to health and safety, such as needing to have an injection or having to hold an adult's hand when crossing the road.

The term 'good touch' can be confusing because it implies that some types of touching are inherently good, regardless of the context or the relationship between the people involved. For example, a hug from a trusted family member or friend might be considered a 'good touch', but if that same person were to touch a child's private parts (outside of expected, pre-arranged caregiving), it would be inappropriate and potentially abusive. Using the term 'good touch' can also make it difficult for children to understand that they have the right to say no to any type of touching that makes them uncomfortable, even if it is from someone they know and trust.

(Left) Figure 7.3: Early warning signs
Source: Educate2Empower (n.d.)

A parent once reported to me that after she had purchased Jayneen Sanders' excellent body safety book, *My Body! What I Say Goes!*, and explained the body safety rules to her seven-year-old, the child was able to verbalise that she felt uncomfortable with the way a particular family member always greeted her – the way he rubbed her back. The family member was a known perpetrator of past sexual abuse in the family. The parent then communicated to all of the family members that her children were learning body safety and no longer had to greet adults if they didn't want to.

Some people may be shocked by this story – that a known perpetrator was free to continue to interact with his family and children – but the statistics are telling. Perpetrators can be anywhere; they are not all in jail or away from children. Many are not even discovered or charged. According to the parent, this adult's assaulting has never been reported.

Similarly, the term 'bad touch' can be misleading because it suggests that some types of touching are always bad or harmful. However, there may be situations where physical contact is necessary for medical or hygiene reasons, such as during a healthcare examination or when helping a child with toileting. In these cases, it is important for children to understand that while the touching may feel bad, uncomfortable or embarrassing, it is not abusive, harmful or unsafe.

 Conversation starters

- A bigger kid or adult should never tell you to keep a secret that gives you your early warning signs. Happy surprises, like a birthday present, are always good, because they will always be talked about — but a secret that you are told to never tell is not okay.

Respect, consent and sexual violence

- You can say to your kinder friends: I am the boss of my body! Or stop it, I don't like it! What else can you say when you don't want a hug?
- It's okay to touch your own body parts. Who else can touch that part of your body, and why?
- You can ask us anything, even if you think it is rude, or bad, or a swear word. I'd rather you check with us. We will always tell you the truth and you won't get in trouble.

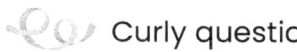 Curly questions

What are privates?

'Privates' is a name used to describe people's genitals at the front and bottom/anus at the back. It can also include breasts and nipples and your mouth. Genitals are the body parts between people's legs at the front. They include the vulva, clitoris, vagina, penis, scrotum and testicles.

Your private parts are for you only, unless you need help with care/washing/medical help/hygiene and one of your trusted adults knows about it, such as Pop, Aunty Lisa or Teacher Sam.

Who can touch my privates?

When you need help to wipe your bottom, to clean your vulva/penis or to put medicine/cream on this area, you can ask: Nonna, the babysitter, the kindy teachers, or Mumma and I to help you. No-one else should touch your private parts because they are just for you. Sometimes we will say it's okay for other adults to help you, like the doctor or Taylor's parents when you have a play date, as long as one of your trusted adults knows about it.

Why are you touching the baby's privates?

I have to touch their vulva/penis/bottom to clean it, to keep it healthy, and I'm telling them about it so they know why.

I am one of their trusted adults and their other trusted adults know that I need to do this to keep them healthy.

I don't like it when Sam kisses and hugs me at kinder.

Sam has forgotten that we all have a body boundary, we call our body bubble. It's our personal space around our body, isn't it? You don't have to like it, especially if your body bubble is being broken. You can say, 'Stop! I don't like it!' in a loud voice and then tell an adult.

Mum, where is your penis?

Physical female bodies don't have a penis, they have a vulva (consider adding clitoris) on the outside and a vagina on the inside.

Daddy, why don't you have boobies?

Good question! All bodies have breast tissue and we all have nipples too.

The type of bodies that have ovaries and a uterus can grow babies. The breasts on those bodies are designed to be larger so that they can make milk to feed the baby. I have testicles, not ovaries.

Why do boys stand up to do wee?

Where the wee/urine comes out of the body is different for different types of bodies.

Bodies with a vulva have a little hole at the top of the vulva, called the urethral opening, above the vagina opening. The wee comes out of that, so it's easier to sit on the toilet.

Bodies with a penis have a little hole out of the top of the penis (the urethral opening) where the wee comes out. Those people can stand up and hold the penis and point it towards the toilet, or they can also sit down too.

Why do some adults do sexual things with kids?

Some adults and other (bigger) kids break the important rules about body safety and sexual behaviour. This is very wrong, and especially the adults know that it is wrong. That's why you might hear about it on the news: it is illegal.

If a kid or an adult does something to you or says something (online or in person) that gives you your early warning signs, you must tell someone in your safety network — especially if they touch your body in your private area or show you pictures of private parts. You can tell us anything.

What is rape?

Sometimes one person uses power over another person by forcing them to do something. Sometimes this is done using sex. A person forces the other person to do sexual things. It is illegal and it is never okay.

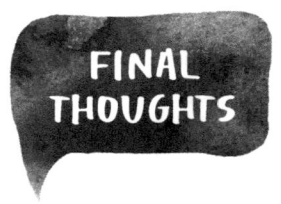

Top 20 tips

My tag line is 'Let's get started, it's easier than you think.' You are already well on your way, having accessed this book. It's a great start and commitment to providing your child with the best opportunity for a fulfilling and safe journey through life.

At the parent sessions I facilitate I always ask the audience to reflect on and tell us about their upbringing: how they learned about sex, sexuality and related topics. The overwhelming majority recount very poor education from school, and conversations at home that were not much better – if they were had at all. Imagine in years to come when your children, by then adults, attend a similar parent session, and they can recount that they had multiple, ongoing, open conversations with their parents (you) that provided them with useful information. They will hopefully say that not only did it shape and inform their safe, healthy and happy sexuality journey and script for their life, but that what they learned helps them to parent their own children (your grandchildren).

The power for that to happen rests with you. Right now. We must break the cycle of the past; the inadequate experience most of us were subject to needs to stop here. This generation of children deserves better. With the evidence we have that age-appropriate, comprehensive, accurate sexuality education protects children from harm, let alone all the positive pleasurable benefits it brings, I actually think it is neglectful for us to continue to ignore these topics. So, thanks for being here.

I'll leave you with my 20 top tips as a cheat sheet you can quickly flick through when you need a nudge to have some conversations, harness teachable moments and be that askable and tellable parent about all things human sexuality, respectful relationships and consent. Ideally you'll bring a positive and joyful, engaging approach to these conversations with your precious kids. Start now. Talking the talk is about having many conversations. Remove your adult layers of 'stuff' in your mind and keep it simple. The benefits outweigh your discomfort, and practise makes perfect. Good luck!

1. Just get started

Be brave and get started. It's never too late (or too early) to start.

Don't worry about giving a child too much information: they will tune out if they are not ready to hear what you're saying. Use the ages and stages guide in chapter 2 to guide you, and pay attention to what your child's level of development is. Ask questions and listen to their everyday comments and conversations.

Use teachable moments (they are everywhere) to get started, or buy some books to read with your child.

Remember, this is not just one 'big talk' – it is many, many conversations over the years of your child's upbringing. It's about building a relationship with your child so that you are the one they trust to give them the information they need.

2. Be the first person to explain each topic to your child

Ask yourself, when do you need to have a conversation with your child to make sure you get in first with each topic – before other kids, other adults, the media, the internet or advertising?

3. Remember it's about more than just sexual encounters

You are responsible for teaching your child about human sexuality and all the interesting topics, diversity and unique experiences to celebrate.

4. Know that the benefits outweigh your discomfort

Your tone of voice is more important than the words you say. Give the vibe that it's okay to talk about these topics. Don't be too serious – especially with older kids. Keeping the lines of communication open is more important than teaching a lesson at every opportunity. Even if you are shocked or angry, it's important to avoid placing barriers between you and your child.

Try to respond positively. It's also okay to say you are a bit embarrassed because you are not used to talking about these topics – no-one ever spoke to you about them when you were young, but you want your child to have a better experience.

5. Let go of your own history

We need to step outside of our own sexual journey, experiences and thoughts when we're teaching our kids about human sexuality – especially if our past has given us a negative attitude towards sex and sexuality.

Every adult mind includes layer upon layer of its own sexual story. Strip these layers back (excuse the pun!): they are not relevant or useful to the simple questions your children are asking or the information that you need to give them.

Remember, young children's questions are mostly not sexual – they do not experience sexual desire or intent before puberty.

6. Be the askable and tellable parent they need you to be

Give your kids limitless permission to ask you anything. Encourage their questions so they know you are their touchstone for information. Tell them: 'You can ask us anything, even if you think it is rude, offensive or a swear word. You won't get in trouble.'

7. Be sexuality positive

Have a positive and open attitude towards human sexuality rather than being focused on fear and danger.

Learning about human sexuality is not dangerous, disgusting, shameful or taboo. On the contrary, evidence clearly shows that kids make better decisions and are healthier and happier when they have had many open, positive conversations with their parents and other adults, such as teachers, carers and health professionals.

8. Remember you are responsible for your children's sexual health, safety and wellbeing

Talking about sexuality is just as important as giving your kids other health and safety messages such as water safety, healthy eating and road safety.

9. Keep it simple but accurate

Use accurate names for body parts, provide accurate descriptions of the different types of intimate experiences that humans can experience, and tell the truth. Information is empowering. Remember, education is not 'permission' and is not harmful, especially when you add in your family values and expectations along the way.

10. Frame your family discussions

Outline the parameters of your family discussions. Make sure your kids know that home is a safe place for any questions and discussion.

Explain to them that not all families are as safe and open about these conversations and it is not their job to teach other children – it is those children's parents' job.

Tell them: 'This is not a public topic and not really one to openly discuss at school, especially as some kids' parents might not have talked to them yet.'

11. Talk in the car or while doing the dishes

It's less confronting for you both as you are facing away from each other. Also, in the car, they are a 'captive' audience! ☺

12. Buy yourself time when faced with challenging questions

Positively reinforce to your child that you are happy they asked such a great question, then ask them what they already know to buy yourself time to formulate your response. You could say something like, 'That is a great question – I am glad you asked me that. How did you hear about it?' or, 'Thanks for asking me that question. Tell me, what do you already know about it?' or, 'That's a really important question, I'm glad you asked. What made you think about that?'

13. Expect sexuality conversations

Sexuality development and behaviour is typical for children and to be expected. There are different expectations for different ages and stages. If you are open to the idea that learning about human sexuality is learning about being human at any age, you can then expect that these topics and questions will come up – and when they do, you can respond positively.

14. Practise, practise, practise

Knowing what to say can be hard, but remember you don't have to be perfect. Saying something is better than nothing!

Try saying the words out loud to another adult. Say 'vulva' to yourself when you see a Volvo car out driving. Talking about sexual and reproductive body parts and functions takes a bit of getting used to, especially when most parents never received adequate sexuality education themselves.

15. Use teachable moments — they are everywhere

Think advertising billboards, commercial radio and TV and computer games. Listen to your kids' favourite songs in the car and call out disrespectful song lyrics on the radio.

Teachable moments can also be positive. For example, while your child is playing their favourite game, you might say something like: 'I love that in Fortnite the characters' outfits don't focus on showing cleavage and other body parts in a sexy way. The feminine costumes look as strong and awesome as the masculine costumes. What do you think?'

16. Use teachable statements

A short accurate statement of information or of your values and expectations can be a great way to get a message across.

You don't always have to have two-way conversations to educate your child. Even if they seem not to be interested or don't want to hear it from you, they are still listening. Saying a statement when you get an opportunity can be enough.

Try something like: 'It's good to hear a condom ad on the radio. It's an important message for people to know that a condom needs to be used every time someone engages in a penetrative sexual activity (or sexy times that involve a penis or shared dildo).'

17. Pick your battles — you can't call out everything

While teachable moments are everywhere, avoid commenting on every single thing. When you have decided to deliver a message, make it effective by ensuring the timing is right – such as when you and the kids are calm and relaxed and there is a vibe of open communication.

18. Be honest

It's a good teaching opportunity to tell your kids you are finding this difficult. The topic of sex and sexuality has been shrouded in mystery and taboo for generations. To change this takes a lot of adjustment.

Explain that in the past people have been discouraged to talk about sex and that it was seen as a bad thing. But we now know that the more we talk about these topics and understand that they are a normal and awesome part of being human, the better experiences people have and the healthier and happier everyone can be.

You can say something like: 'No-one ever spoke to me about this, so I'm a bit shy and embarrassed – bear with me while I find the best words to explain it to you.'

Just keep talking – it is great role modelling that you discuss difficult things. Your children will learn from you that they, too, can talk about hard things when they are learning to communicate with partners in the future.

19. It's okay not to answer right away

Don't rush your response if you are not sure about it. It's okay to say, 'I'd like to look that up so I can answer your question the best I can – I'll get back to you.' This also helps you test the waters and observe their reaction before expanding and adding more detail.

20. Don't stop parenting too early

Our kids need our support, advice and listening skills on these topics, especially navigating relationships, well into their late teens and early 20s. Don't withdraw too soon.

Lastly, as I always say: *let's get started, it's easier than you think!*

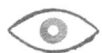 Self-reflection

What were your key takeaways from reading this book? Write down your insights and ideas to improve your conversations with your kids.

Final thoughts: top 20 tips

SEXUALITY CONVERSATION STARTERS

Here are some conversation prompts and ideas to adapt to your style for discussions with your child as they grow from young children to adults.

Younger kids

- What do you think that means?
- Remember when you asked me about …
- You can say to your kinder friends: I am the boss of my body! What else can you say when you don't want a hug?
- It's okay to touch your own body parts. Who else can touch that part of your body, and why? (Caregiving only.)
- I know that it feels good to touch your private area/vulva/penis – where is a private place you can go to do that? (Bedroom.)
- You can ask us anything, even if you think it is rude, or bad, or a swear word, I'd rather you check with us. We will always tell you the truth and you won't get in trouble.
- Your body is so amazing. It can … When you grow up, what changes do you think will happen?

- No, these eggs don't have a chick in them, because they were not fertilised – the chickens were not with a rooster. Let me explain how eggs get fertilised. Did you know humans have eggs too?

- Thanks for asking questions. I like it when you ask me things.

- Look at that amazing strong pregnant person. That reminds me, we haven't talked about the incredible way babies are made – what do you know about it?

- Talking about funny words, there is a strange but really important word we need to talk about. Have you ever heard of the word 'sex'?

- Wow! Those teenagers are tall. What else do you notice about them that's different from being a younger kid?

- Remember, it isn't your job to teach this to other kids – that it is the job of the adults who look after those kids. You can ask us anything, but not all families have the open chats that we have, so this is not a conversation to share in the playground.

Older kids

- You might have been waiting for me to bring this up – sorry it has taken me so long.

- We talked about this the other day but there is a bit more to it that I need to cover with you.

- It's time we had a chat about …

- Do you have any questions about what you're feeling or the changes you're going through?

- I feel a little uncomfortable, and you might too, which is normal, but this is really important.

- It's okay to feel embarrassed. Keep talking and it will get easier.
- It seems like you don't want to talk about this right now, and that's okay. Can you let me know a time that might suit you better?
- I think you're mature enough to talk about this now.
- I'm glad I saw this. You are not in trouble but you do need some help and advice so you might make different decisions next time.
- At this age everyone is developing at different rates, ages and levels.
- Does your new phone take good photos? Do you know what a digital footprint is?
- Last year of primary school for you! I remember feeling sad to leave my friends for high school. How about you?
- I was reading that the age you're at is good and bad because you still get to have all the fun of a kid but also have to do more independent 'teenager' things at the same time, like washing your own clothes. What will you miss about being a kid?

Oldest kids

- I just need five minutes of your time. There is something really important that you need to hear from us. You don't have to respond if you don't want to. Is now a good time?
- This bit is important so I'm happy that you're interested.
- It seems like you don't want to talk about this right now, and that's okay. If you ever have any questions, you can ask me.

- There is a really important topic we have not talked about before. It's something that is super important. You can have a think about it and get back to me. Here are the basics …

- I just read this really interesting fact. Can you guess the two most important parts of the body to make bodies feel awesome when people are being intimate/sexual? It's not what you'd expect! (Answer: brain and skin; go on to talk about outercourse and pleasure.)

- Actually that show is not very accurate … pleasure is the main reason people have sexual experiences.

- Yep, but 'sex' means heaps of different things. What do you think most people think it means?

- What does 'hook up' mean among your friends?

- Do you think your friends have had sexual experiences?

- How many hook-ups happen at the parties you go to?

- You and I might have different ideas about this topic and that's okay, but let's hear each other's points of view.

- Help me make up my mind on this … what is your opinion?

- Your reaction shows me you know something about this already …

- Is there more to it than that?

- That person is really obsessed with their bum/hair … Isn't it a shame our society puts so much pressure on us all to look a certain way? Do you feel that pressure?

- What about their brain/personality/feelings/opinions?

- What do kids at school talk about when it comes to the topic of porn?

- Have you and your partner talked about what you are comfortable doing sexually/as your relationship progresses?
- When those things happen at a party do you think people are in a position to give ongoing, freely given agreement/consent?
- What experiences have kids at school had with seeing porn?
- What percentage of your friends do you think have seen porn?
- Some people your age come across porn. Is this something that's happening at your school?
- Do you think most people are fully into that stuff?
- How would you describe people's options for feeling comfortable, private and able to be fully into it if it's happening at a party?
- Do you ever wonder if one of your friends has made a risky choice with a partner?
- It's hard to trust your own judgement/gut feelings when someone is trying to convince you to do something you're not sure about. Does that happen in your group of friends?
- Intimacy and sexual stuff is pretty complex. What do you think is the most confusing part that kids at school need information about?
- That's a great question. I'm glad you asked me about that. It reminds me to ask you about …
- Oh good question, I've been meaning to tell you about that. While we are at it, I need to talk to you about …
- Do you know anyone from the LGBTIQA+ community?
- I don't know the answer to that, but I'll find out and tell you what I learn.

- I think I'll also look up the latest contraception recommendations – it's probably something we need to chat about and help you sort out.
- What videos or articles have you seen that mention porn or sex?
- Do you have questions about what you've seen on the internet or heard people say?
- There are a few key things you have to learn before you start having relationships and dating.
- The legal age of consent for penetrative sex is 16 and over and there are some pretty good reasons for this. What are your thoughts about it?
- Kissing that person without asking is not okay. Coercion is not okay, ever. If someone says no, then it is no. What do you think about this TV show promoting this?
- Is your school a safe place for people who are LGBTIQA+?
- New research says being same-gender-attracted is more common than previously thought. I'm glad we are acknowledging and celebrating people's differences. What do you think?
- Actually that show is unrealistic … sexual experiences are awesome and pleasurable when both people are completely 'into it', not one coercing another.
- Negotiating a mutually enjoyable activity to do together will mean you both have the best experience. What could you say to check they are keen on it?

Resources

Vanessa Hamilton
Talking the Talk Healthy Sexuality Education:
www.talkingthetalksexed.com.au

Sexual development
Raising Children:
https://raisingchildren.net.au/search?query=sexuality%20sexual%20development

National Center on the Sexual Behavior of Youth:
https://www.ncsby.org/content/childhood-sexual-development

Puberty
Raising Children:
https://raisingchildren.net.au/pre-teens/development/puberty-sexual-development/physical-changes-in-puberty

Human sexuality diversity
Minus 18:
www.minus18.org.au/resources/lgbtiq+-inclusive-language-guide

Rainbow Families:
www.rainbowfamilies.com.au

Australian Institute of Family Studies LGBTIQA+ Glossary:
https://aifs.gov.au/sites/default/files/publication-documents/22-02_rs_lgbtiqa_glossary_of_common_terms_0.pdf

Pornography

Culture Reframed:
www.culturereframed.org

It's Time we Talked:
http://itstimewetalked.com

Safe4Kids pornography education books:
https://safe4kids.com.au/product-category/books/

Childhood sexual abuse

Australian Government:
aifs.gov.au/resources/practice-guides/responding-children-and-young-peoples-disclosures-abuse

aifs.gov.au/resources/policy-and-practice-papers/what-child-abuse-and-neglect

Grace Tame:
www.youtube.com/watch?v=tYK4r7zNAdU
www.mamamia.com.au/grace-tame-signs-of-grooming/

Educate2Empower body safety posters:
https://e2epublishing.info/posters

Operation KidSafe: A detective's guide to child abuse prevention (book), Kristi McVee, 2022

Online safety

Australian Centre to Counter Child Exploitation:
www.accce.gov.au/help-and-support/preventing-online-child-sexual-exploitation

Youth Law Australia:
http://yla.org.au

eSafety Commissioner:
www.esafety.gov.au

Take It Down:
http://takeitdown.ncmec.org

Inform & Empower Digital Safety & Wellbeing:
www.informandempower.com.au

Cyber Safety Project:
https://cybersafetyproject.com.au

Consent

Kit and Arlo Find a Way:
https://shop.acer.org/kit-and-arlo-find-a-way.html
www.talkingthetalksexed.com.au/kit-and-arlo

Help and support for adults

Raising Children:
https://raisingchildren.net.au/grown-ups/services-support/about-services-support/helplines

ParentTV:
https://parenttv.com

Help and support for children

Kids Helpline:
https://kidshelpline.com.au

Sexual health education evidence and examples

UNESCO:
https://unesdoc.unesco.org/ark:/48223/pf0000260770

Government of Western Australia:
https://gdhr.wa.gov.au/resources/guidelines/western-australian

References

ACCCE (2022) *Online blackmail and sexual extortion response kit*, accessed 22 May 2023. https://www.accce.gov.au/sites/default/files/2022-06/June%202022%20-%20Online%20blackmail%20and%20sexual%20extortion%20response%20kit.pdf

ACCCE (2023) 'AFP records spike in financial sextortion reports over the school holidays', accessed 22 May 2023. https://www.accce.gov.au/news-and-media/media-release/afp-records-spike-financial-sextortion-reports-over-school-holidays

Armstrong C (2021) 'LGBT+ history month: forgotten figures who challenged gender expression and identity centuries ago', *The Conversation*, accessed 18 June. https://theconversation.com/lgbt-history-month-forgotten-figures-who-challenged-gender-expression-and-identity-centuries-ago-153815

Aubusson K (2022) 'One in 18 babies conceived by IVF but success can depend on choice of clinic', *The Sydney Morning Herald*, accessed 18 June 2023. https://www.smh.com.au/national/one-in-18-babies-conceived-by-ivf-but-success-can-depend-on-choice-of-clinic-20221014-p5bpwd.html

Australian Child Maltreatment Study (2023), accessed 23 May 2023. https://www.acms.au/

Australian Government (2017) *Problem sexual behaviours and sexually abusive behaviours in Australian children and young people*, accessed 17 June 2023. https://aifs.gov.au/resources/policy-and-practice-papers/problem-sexual-behaviours-and-sexually-abusive-behaviours

Australian Government (2018) 'What is child abuse and neglect?', accessed 23 May 2023. https://aifs.gov.au/resources/policy-and-practice-papers/what-child-abuse-and-neglect

Australian Government (2020) *Sexual assault in Australia*, accessed 22 May 2023. https://www.aihw.gov.au/reports/domestic-violence/sexual-assault-in-australia/contents/summary

Australian Government (2022a) *LGBTIQA+ glossary of common terms*, accessed 17 June 2023. https://aifs.gov.au/sites/default/files/publication-documents/22-02_rs_lgbtiqa_glossary_of_common_terms_0.pdf

Australian Government (2022b) 'Child abuse and neglect', accessed 17 June 2023. https://www.aihw.gov.au/reports/children-youth/australias-children/contents/justice-and-safety/child-abuse-and-neglect

Australian Government (2023a) 'Bring Up Respect', accessed 22 May 2023. https://www.respect.gov.au/

Australian Government (2023b) *The Conversation Guide*, accessed 18 May 2023. https://www.respect.gov.au/resources/talking-about-respect/

Australian Human Rights Commission (n.d.) 'Terminology: LBBTIQ+', accessed 18 June 2023. https://humanrights.gov.au/our-work/lgbti/terminology

Baron D (2018) 'A brief history of singular "they"', *Oxford English Dictionary* blog, accessed 17 June 2023. https://public.oed.com/blog/a-brief-history-of-singular-they/

BBC News (2019) 'A brief history of gender neutral pronouns', accessed 17 June 2023. https://www.bbc.com/news/newsbeat-49754930

Bonitatibus S (2023) 'Key Issues Facing People With Intersex Traits', Center for American Progress, accessed 18 June 2023. https://www.americanprogress.org/article/key-issues-facing-people-intersex-traits/

Bravehearts Foundation (n.d.) 'What is Grooming?', accessed 23 May 2023. https://bravehearts.org.au/about-child-sexual-abuse/what-is-grooming/

Children's Commissioner (2023) *'A lot of it is actually just abuse': Young people and pornography*, accessed 22 May 2023. https://assets.childrenscommissioner.gov.uk/wpuploads/2023/02/cc-a-lot-of-it-is-actually-just-abuse-young-people-and-pornography-updated.pdf

Cottier C (2021) 'People Have Used They/Them as Singular Pronouns for Hundreds of Years', Discover, accessed 17 June 2023. https://www.discovermagazine.com/mind/people-have-used-they-them-as-singular-pronouns-for-hundreds-of-years

Culture Reframed (2023) 'A New Tool to Support Porn-Critical Sex Education', accessed 18 June 2023. https://www.culturereframed.org/a-new-tool-to-support-porn-critical-sex-education/

Diemer K (2015) 'ABS Personal Safety Survey: Additional analysis on relationship and sex of perpetrator', University of Melbourne.

Educate2Empower (n.d.) 'Resources: Posters', accessed 23 May 2023. https://e2epublishing.info/posters

eSafety Commissioner (n.d.) 'Sexting and sending nudes', accessed 18 June 2023. https://www.esafety.gov.au/key-issues/staying-safe/sending-nudes-sexting

eSafety Commissioner (25 May 2023) 'Sexual extortion and child abuse reports almost triple', accessed 31 July 2023. https://www.esafety.gov.au/newsroom/media-releases/sexual-extortion-and-child-abuse-reports-almost-triple

Fisher C et al. (1983) 'Patterns of female sexual arousal during sleep and waking: Vaginal utgers-conductance studies', *Archives of Sexual Behavior*, 12(2):97-122.

Fisher C et al. (2019) *6th National Survey of Australian Secondary Students and Sexual Health 2018*, Australian Research Centre in Sex, Health & Society, La Trobe University.

Flood M (2017) 'Engaging men in violence prevention: Key resources', XY, accessed 22 May 2023. https://xyonline.net/content/engaging-men-violence-prevention-key-resources

Ford J et al. (2021) 'The World Association for Sexual Health's Declaration on Sexual Pleasure: A Technical Guide', *International Journal of Sexual Health*, 33(4):612-642.

Frederick DA, John HKS and Garcia JR et al. (2018) 'Differences in Orgasm Frequency Among Gay, Lesbian, Bisexual, and Heterosexual Men and Women in a U.S. National Sample', *Archives of Sexual Behavior*, 47:273-288.

Government of Canada (2023) 'The human rights of lesbian, gay, bisexual, transgender, queer, 2-spirit and intersex persons', accessed 17 June 2023. https://www.international.gc.ca/world-monde/issues_development-enjeux_developpement/human_rights-droits_homme/rights_lgbti-droits_lgbti.aspx?lang=eng

Government of Western Australia (n.d. a) 'Ages and stages', Talk soon. Talk often., accessed 5 July 2023. https://tsto.gdhr.wa.gov.au/ages-and-stages/birth-to-2-years

Government of Western Australia (n.d. b) 'Child sexual abuse', Talk soon. Talk often., accessed 23 May 2023. https://tsto.gdhr.wa.gov.au/keeping-children-safe/sexual-abuse

Government of Western Australia Department of Health (2023) 'Relationships and sexuality education', accessed 17 May 2023. https://gdhr.wa.gov.au/guides/teaching-rse

Healthychildren.org (2022) 'Teen Suicide Risk: What Parents Should Know', accessed 17 June 2023. https://www.healthychildren.org/English/health-issues/conditions/emotional-problems/Pages/which-kids-are-at-highest-risk-for-suicide.aspx

Hendriks J et al. (2023) 'Support for school-based relationships and sexual health education: a national survey of Australian parents', *Sex Education*, 21 March 2023.

Herbenick D et al. (2018) 'Women's Experiences With Genital Touching, Sexual Pleasure, and Orgasm: Results From a U.S. Probability Sample of Women Ages 18 to 94', *Journal of Sex & Marital Therapy*, 44(2):201-12.

References

Higgins D (2023) 'Major study reveals two-thirds of people who suffer childhood maltreatment suffer more than one kind', *The Conversation*, accessed 23 May 2023. https://theconversation-com.cdn.ampproject.org/c/s/theconversation.com/amp/major-study-reveals-two-thirds-of-people-who-suffer-childhood-maltreatment-suffer-more-than-one-kind-202033

Hill A et al. (2021a) *Private Lives 3: The health and wellbeing of LGBTQ people in Victoria: Victoria summary report*, Australian Research Centre in Sex, Health and Society, La Trobe University.

Hill A et al. (2021b) *Writing Themselves In 4*, Australian Research Centre in Sex, Health and Society, La Trobe University, accessed 17 June 2023. https://www.latrobe.edu.au/__data/assets/pdf_file/0010/1198945/Writing-Themselves-In-4-National-report.pdf

Hillier L et al. (2010) *Writing Themselves In 3*, Australian Research Centre in Sex, Health and Society, La Trobe University, accessed 16 June 2023. https://www.latrobe.edu.au/arcshs/documents/arcshs-research-publications/Wti3.pdf

Historic England (n.d.) 'Trans and Gender-Nonconforming Histories', accessed 18 June 2023. https://historicengland.org.uk/research/inclusive-heritage/lgbtq-heritage-project/trans-and-gender-nonconforming-histories/

Intersex Human Rights Australia (2013) 'What is intersex?', accessed 18 June 2023. https://ihra.org.au/18106/what-is-intersex/

Intersex Human Rights Australia (2019) 'Intersex population figures', accessed 18 May 2023. https://ihra.org.au/16601/intersex-numbers/

Jade E Newman JE, Paul RC and Chambers GM (2022) *Assisted reproductive technology in Australia and New Zealand 2020*, The University of New South Wales, accessed 16 June 2023. https://npesu.unsw.edu.au/sites/default/files/npesu/data_collection/Assisted%20Reproductive%20Technology%20in%20Australia%20and%20New%20Zealand%202020.pdf

Jepsten B (2021) 'In 2017, Grace Tame looked up the word "grooming". She was both validated and horrified', Mamamia, accessed 17 June 2023. https://www.mamamia.com.au/grace-tame-signs-of-grooming/

Laguna I and Hamilton V (2022) *Kit and Arlo Find a Way: Teaching consent to 8-12 year olds*, ACER Press.

Lehmiller J (2019) 'How Often Do Women Orgasm During Sex?', Kinsey Institute, accessed 16 June 2023. https://blogs.iu.edu/kinseyinstitute/2019/01/24/how-often-do-women-orgasm-during-sex/

LGBTIQA+ Health Australia (2021) *Snapshot of Mental Health and Suicide Prevention Statistics For LGBTIQ+ People*, accessed 17 June 2023. https://assets.nationbuilder.com/lgbtihealth/pages/549/attachments/original/1648014801/24.10.21_Snapshot_of_MHSP_Statistics_for_LGBTIQ__People_-_Revised.pdf?1648014801

LibreTexts (n.d.) '26.5E: Vagina', accessed 16 June 2023. https://med.libretexts.org/Bookshelves/Anatomy_and_Physiology/Anatomy_and_Physiology_(Boundless)/26%3A_The_Reproductive_System/26.5%3A_The_Female_Reproductive_System/26.5E%3A_Vagina

Lucke J and Taft A (2019) 'Understanding why women have abortions', La Trobe University, accessed 29 June 2023. https://www.latrobe.edu.au/news/articles/2019/opinion/understanding-why-women-have-abortions

Marson K (2022) *Legitimate Sexpectations: The power of sex-ed*, Scribe.

McKay A and Bissell M (2020) *Sexual health education in the schools: Questions & Answers* (3rd ed.), Sex Information and Education Council of Canada (SIECCAN).

Midsumma festival (n.d.) Inclusive Language Guide, accessed 18 June 2023. https://www.midsumma.org.au/media/ooyffkap/inclusive_language_guide_171220.pdf

Minus18 (n.d.) *LGBTIQ+ Inclusive Language Guide*, accessed 18 June 2023. https://www.minus18.org.au/resources/lgbtiq+-inclusive-language-guide

Mount Sinai Adolescent Health Center (2019) 'You Asked It: What are Wet Dreams?', Mount Sinai Adolescent Health Center: Teen Health Care, accessed 18 June 2023. https://www.teenhealthcare.org/blog/you-asked-it-what-are-wet-dreams/

MRKH Australia (n.d.) 'About MRKH', accessed 29 June 2023. https://www.mrkhaustralia.org/about-mrkh

Murray L, Thomas C, McGovern A, Milivojevic, S (2015) *Sexting among young people: Perceptions and practices*, Australian Institute of Criminology, 1836-2206, accessed 18 June 2023. https://www.aic.gov.au/publications/tandi/tandi508

National Academies of Sciences, Engineering, and Medicine (2020) *Understanding the Well-Being of LGBTQI+ Populations*, The National Academies Press.

National Center on the Sexual Behavior of Youth (n.d.) 'Childhood Sexual Development', accessed 18 June 2023. https://www.ncsby.org/content/childhood-sexual-development

NSW Government (n.d.) *Talking About It*, accessed 5 July 2023. https://www.health.nsw.gov.au/parvan/hsb/Documents/talking-about-it.pdf

Nunn L (creator) (2021) *Sex Education* [television program] (season 3), Netflix.

OECD (2019) *Educating 21st Century Children: Emotional Well-being in the Digital Age*, accessed 22 May 2023. https://www.oecd-ilibrary.org/sites/71b7058a-en/index.html?itemId=/content/component/71b7058a-en

Office of the United Nations High Commissioner for Human Rights (OHCHR) (n.d.) 'Background Note on Human Rights Violations against Intersex People', accessed 18 June 2023. https://www.ohchr.org/en/documents/tools-and-resources/background-note-human-rights-violations-against-intersex-people

Opie, T (2022) What parents need to know about 'sending nudes' *SBS Voices*, accessed 18 June 2023. https://www.sbs.com.au/topics/voices/relationships/article/2019/07/12/what-parents-need-know-about-sending-nudes

Our Watch (2020) *Pornography, young people, and preventing violence against women*, accessed 22 May 2023. https://media-cdn.ourwatch.org.au/wp-content/uploads/sites/2/2020/11/20022415/Pornography-young-people-preventing-violence.pdf

Our Watch (2022) *Men in focus practice guide: Addressing masculinities and working with men in the prevention of men's violence against women*, accessed 30 June 2023. https://media-cdn.ourwatch.org.au/wp-content/uploads/sites/2/2022/08/19131630/Men-in-focus-practice-guide-accessible.pdf

Our Watch (2023) 'Change the story', accessed 17 June 2023. https://www.ourwatch.org.au/change-the-story/

Perales F, Ablaza C and Elkin N (2022) 'Exposure to Inclusive Language and Well-Being at Work Among Transgender Employees in Australia', *American Journal of Public Health*, 112(3):482-90.

Pound P et al. (2017) 'What is best practice in sex and relationship education? A synthesis of evidence, including stakeholders' views', *BMJ Open*, 7:e014791.

Power J et al. (2022) *The 7th National Survey of Australian Secondary Students and Sexual Health 2021*, The Australian Research Centre in Sex, Health and Society, La Trobe University.

Rafferty J (2022) 'Gender Identity Development in Children', healthychildren.org, accessed 18 May 2023. https://www.healthychildren.org/English/ages-stages/gradeschool/Pages/Gender-Identity-and-Gender-Confusion-In-Children.aspx

RAINN (n.d.) 'Child Sexual Abuse', accessed 30 June 2023. https://www.rainn.org/articles/child-sexual-abuse

Raising Children Network (n.d.) 'Teens: puberty & sexual development', accessed 2 August 2023. https://raisingchildren.net.au/teens/development/puberty-sexual-development

Raising Children Network (2022) 'Fraternal twins, identical twins and other types of twins', accessed 5 July 2023. https://raisingchildren.net.au/pregnancy/health-wellbeing/twin-pregnancy/twins

References

Raising Children Network (2023) 'Sexting: talking with teenagers', accessed 18 June 2023. https://raisingchildren.net.au/teens/entertainment-technology/pornography-sexting/sexting-teens#what-teenagers-wish-their-parents-knew-about-sexting-nav-title

Ramírez-Villalobos D et al. (2021) 'Delaying sexual onset: outcome of a comprehensive sexuality education initiative for adolescents in public schools', *BMC Public Health*, 21:1439.

Rutgers (2022) *Sexuality education in the Netherlands*, accessed 29 June 2023. https://rutgers.international/resources/sexuality-education-in-the-netherlands/

Rutgers (n.d.) 'Dutch attitudes and approaches to sexuality', accessed 16 June 2023. https://rutgers.international/about-rutgers/dutch-attitudes-and-approaches-to-sexuality

Sanders J (2016) *My Body! What I Say Goes!*, Educate2Empower Publishing.

Sex Information & Education Council of Canada (2023) '2SLGBTQINA+ Inclusive Sexual Health Education: SIECCAN Issue BRIEF', accessed 18 June 2023. https://www.sieccan.org/post/2slgbtqina-inclusive-sexual-health-education-sieccan-issue-brief

Sexual Health Victoria (2022) 'LGBTQIA+ Inclusive Language Guide', accessed 18 June 2023. https://shvic.org.au/assets/resources/SHV_InclusiveLangugeGuide_Public.pdf

Sharman L, Douglas H and Fitzgerald R (n.d.), *Violence Deaths Involving Fatal and Non-Fatal Strangulation in Queensland*, Queensland Courts, accessed 29 June 2023. https://www.courts.qld.gov.au/__data/assets/pdf_file/0006/698586/review-of-dv-deaths-involving-fatal-and-non-fatal-strangulation-in-queensland.pdf

Simpson G (2003) *You and Me: A guide to sex and sexuality after a traumatic brain injury*, 2nd edn.

Tame G (2021) 'The Six Stages Of Sexual Grooming Explained By Grace Tame' [video], 10 News First, YouTube, accessed 17 June 2023. https://www.youtube.com/watch?v=tYK4r7zNAdU

The National Child Traumatic Stress Network in Partnership with NCSBY (2009) 'Sexual Development and Behavior in Children: Information for Parents and Caregivers', accessed 18 June 2023. https://www.ncsby.org/sites/default/files/NCTSN%20NCSBY%20sexualdevelopmentandbehavior%202009.pdf

Tomazin F and Prytz A (3 May 2021) 'It's a "man's problem", so how do we talk to boys about sexual harassment?', The Age, accessed 22 May 2023. https://www.theage.com.au/national/it-s-a-man-s-problem-so-how-do-we-talk-to-boys-about-sexual-harassment-20210429-p57nmo.html

TransHub (n.d.) 'Trans-affirming clinical language guide', accessed 18 June 2023. https://az659834.vo.msecnd.net/eventsairaueprod/production-ashm-public/1e128ca739ee481a8c30d27f1b257f12

True Relationships and Reproductive Health (n.d.) *Traffic Lights® for professionals*, accessed 18 June 2023. https://www.true.org.au/education/programs-resources/for-schools-teachers/traffic-lights-for-professionals

True Relationships and Reproductive Health (2019) *Traffic Lights Sexual behaviours in children and young people: A guide to identify, understand and respond to sexual behaviours*, Brisbane, Queensland.

UNESCO (2018) *International technical guidance on sexuality education: An evidence-informed approach*, 2nd edn, accessed 17 May 2023. https://unesdoc.unesco.org/ark:/48223/pf0000260770

University of California (2019) 'Exploring the history of gender expression', accessed 18 May 2023. https://link.ucop.edu/2019/10/14/exploring-the-history-of-gender-expression/

University of Melbourne (n.d.) 'Diverse sexuality, sex and gender (LGBTIQA+)', accessed 29 June 2023. https://services.unimelb.edu.au/counsel/resources/relationships/diverse-sexuality-sex-and-gender-lgbtiqa

Victorian Assisted Reproductive Treatment Authority (2022) *2022 Annual Report*, accessed 18 June 2023. https://www.varta.org.au/sites/default/files/2022-12/6910%20VARTA_AR2022_188p_final2.pdf

Victorian Government (2021) 'Definitions and key terms', accessed 22 May 2023. https://www.vic.gov.au/pride-our-future-victorias-lgbtiq-strategy-2022-32/definitions-and-key-terms

Victorian Government (2021) 'LGBTIQ+ Inclusive Language Guide', accessed 18 May 2023. https://www.vic.gov.au/inclusive-language-guide

Victorian Government Department of Health (2023) 'Health of people with intersex variations', accessed 18 May 2023. https://www.health.vic.gov.au/populations/health-of-people-with-intersex-variations

World Bank (n.d.) 'Adolescent fertility rate (births per 1,000 women ages 15-19)', accessed 29 June 2023. https://genderdata.worldbank.org/indicators/sp-ado-tfrt/?view=bar&year=2020

World Health Organization (2017) 'Sexual health and its linkages to reproductive health: an operational approach', accessed 17 May 2023. https://apps.who.int/iris/bitstream/handle/10665/258738/9789241512886-eng.pdf

World Health Organization (2023a) 'Sexual and Reproductive Health and Research (SRH)', accessed 17 May 2023. https://www.who.int/teams/sexual-and-reproductive-health-and-research/key-areas-of-work/sexual-health/defining-sexual-health

World Health Organization (2023b) 'Gender and health', accessed 18 May 2023. https://www.who.int/health-topics/gender#tab=tab_1

World Health Organization (2023c) '1 in 6 people globally affected by infertility: WHO', accessed 18 June 2023. https://www.who.int/news/item/04-04-2023-1-in-6-people-globally-affected-by-infertility

About Vanessa

Vanessa Hamilton is a sexuality educator, a mum to three wonderful kids, a partner and a household manager.

Vanessa became a sexual health nurse by chance. In 1993, while backpacking around the world, she accepted a nursing agency shift taking blood tests in a London HIV/AIDS clinic. It was an interesting and equally devastating time to work in sexual health, with the world in the grip of an HIV epidemic.

Upon her return to Australia, Vanessa worked at Melbourne Sexual Health Centre (MSHC) for more than 16 years. She was a clinical sexual and reproductive health nurse, a nursing services manager for five years, and a lecturer and honorary fellow at the University of Melbourne. She then worked at a large tertiary teaching hospital in Melbourne where she supported people with spinal cord injuries, cancer, acquired brain injuries and many other illnesses and injures with their sexual health and wellbeing. Part of her role was to teach doctors, nurses and allied health professionals how to incorporate sexual health into patient and client care.

Vanessa has been a registered nurse for 32 years including more than 25 years working in sexual and reproductive health and education. Her business, Talking the Talk Healthy Sexuality Education, started when she realised talking to her kids about the complexities of human sexuality was even hard for her, let alone what is must be like for other parents! She discovered her sexual health experience had not prepared her for the conversations she needed to have with her children. She decided it was time to do something about the lack of knowledge and confidence among parents and teachers to support children's sexual health, wellbeing and safety.

In 2013 Vanessa delivered her first parent presentation at her children's school. These parent sessions led to schools requesting a contemporary approach to the delivery of their student education, as many external providers they hired were not adequate. This resulted in Vanessa being privileged to teach students from ages five to 21 in schools and universities for more than seven years, as well as continuing to teach parents, educators and health professionals.

Vanessa has presented to tens of thousands of parents, educators, health professionals and students. She has educated in youth detention centres, universities, local councils, schools, kindergartens, hospitals, community health centres and youth services centres in rural, regional and metropolitan areas.

During the pandemic Vanessa created the Talking the Talk Virtual classroom subscription program which continues to be an essential part of her offering. It allows schools and parents to access an online platform of resources and videos, for student education from Foundation to Year 12, matched to the Australian Curriculum, combined with in-person training and support. In 2022 she was fortunate to collaborate with renowned children's author Ingrid Laguna on the book *Kit and Arlo Find a Way*: a page-turning chapter book about consent accompanied by a dedicated digital teaching resource platform.

www.talkingthetalksexed.com.au

Acknowledgements

Firstly, to my three amazing boys: this book is for you. I have learned so much from you all. You were the inspiration for me to write it, to try to make the world a better place for you and your friends to grow up in. Thank you for being so very patient while I created it. The impact on our already full family life was significant. I just hope the book's impact – a brighter future for you and the next generations – makes up for it. It is an absolute privilege to be your mum. I could not be prouder. I love you all more than you can ever imagine.

To my darling husband: we really are the dream team doing life together, with our amazing kids, a needy rescue greyhound and two businesses surviving and thriving. Two books in two years – I'm not sure I would be able to be as patient, tolerant and supportive as you have been while they were being created. I can't thank you enough for your never-ending support. I love you so very much.

To my extended family and friends, always there with messages of support, patiently listening to me complain how challenging this was and providing feedback – even when I would randomly send out a late-night poll for voting on a question about the book. I am very lucky to have you all in my life.

To the people I have come across in my many years working in sexual health and education: you have all taught me so very much. So many inspirational peers and colleagues have and continue to enrich my working and life experience.

Special shout out to Marty McGauran and Carley McGauran from Inform and Empower for encouraging me to create a resource so they could share it with parents – that 'resource' turned into this book.

To the tens of thousands of patients, students and educators who have trusted me to provide them with care and/or education: it has always been a two-way exchange and a privilege to be part of what is a very personal journey in your life. You really have been my teachers as much as I have been yours.

Tess McCabe: it is with so much gratitude that I thank you for creating the opportunity for this book. Thank you for not only sharing in the vision but physically designing the cover and the layout as well!

Alicia Cohen at Amba Press and the team: thank you for the opportunity to get this into the world. I will forever be so very grateful for your unwavering backing, support and encouragement.

Brooke Lyons: you took on an epic editing task, both the nature of the content and my terrible grammar! Your skill and expertise have crafted my 'notes' into a 'real' book that people can actually make sense of. So much gratitude to you.

Finally, and most importantly, to the Talking the Talk team – Joanna Anagnostou, Rebecca Gillie, Emily Mah and Rachelle Deem – for researching, editing, writing, repeat. I could not have done it without your contribution and enthusiasm. It's so very much appreciated.

www.ingramcontent.com/pod-product-compliance
Lightning Source LLC
Chambersburg PA
CBHW050416120526
44590CB00015B/1989